To Erick,
Thank you for the hundreds
of things you have done for
the Foundation For Living Medicine
and me. Your mother
raised you in Love and Light.

Living Medicine

You are a living
example of Living Medicine.
and a great Teacher

Love
Dr. Gladys

2-5-2021

To Andrew
My heart jumped with
joy when you took your
first breath in my Hands
as you were born.

Living Medicine

The world is a better
place as "you" continue to
live your life in Light
and Love.

I Love you
Nami

Dr. Gladys Taylor McGarey with
Dr. Ann McCombs

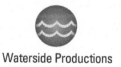

Waterside Productions

Printed in the United States of America

Second Edition First Printing, 2020

ISBN-13: 978-1-949001-93-8 print edition
ISBN-13: 978-1-949001-94-5 ebook edition

Waterside Productions
2055 Oxford Ave
Cardiff, CA 92007
www.waterside.com

Contents

Acknowledgments – Dr. Gladys

Second Edition

I deeply appreciate my parents who, on faith, went to India during WW I— facing untold hardships— and gave me the opportunity to be born in that wondrous land. My siblings filled my life with laughter, tears and great stories. My Indian families and friends enriched my life. I got to watch the healing power of love work in our lives to form bonds which can never be broken. Although poverty and disease were all around us, they did not dominate our thoughts; we simply learned to deal with them as part of Life's lessons. What a rich heritage with which to start life! I see now how those childhood roots laid the groundwork for me to come full circle and evolve the Living Medicine paradigm. I dwell in gratitude for *all* these experiences that made it possible for me to do this.

My six children and their significant others, my ten grandchildren and eight great-grandchildren have each, in their own precious ways, filled my life with meaning and hope.

Through the years, my patients have introduced me to and shared with me the "Physician Within" them, so that we could learn and work together to bring about healing. They have kept me humble, as I watched and worked with the magnificence of the human spirit as it carried people through times of severe pain and sorrow with faith, hope and love. Bobbie Woolf, in particular, has been an extraordinary example of Living Medicine since she was 18 months old. It is she and others like her who have taught me that Life is a mystery to be lived, not a problem to be solved.

My study group partners, who have met in my home weekly since 1957, have shared my prayers, helped me interpret my dreams and study the scriptures. What a blessing!

There are no words to adequately thank Rose Winters (CEO of my Foundation for Living Medicine) enough for her years of faithfully standing by me with loving devotion and *never* wavering in her support of both me and my work throughout the years.

Doris Solbrig typed, proofread and retyped the first edition of this manuscript many times. Without the dedicated, loving assistance, consistent support and meticulous editing skills of my writing partner, Dr. Ann McCombs, there may have never been a *second* edition of this book!

Throughout my whole life I acknowledge the power and grace of the Living God, which has manifested in every moment of my life.

Acknowledgments – Dr. Ann

I wish to first thank my dad and both of my grandmothers for their unwavering belief in and unconditional support of me at significant points in my childhood, teenage and adult years. Without them, and a mother who stood in stark contrast to them, I would never have developed into the person I am today. I am deeply grateful also for the *values* and *principles* they taught me such as integrity, honesty, "failure just shows you what *doesn't* work," "never give up or quit on what really matters to you," "the impossible just takes a little longer," "you're never too old to learn" and "never let the sun set on a quarrel," to name just a few and which have served me well in guiding my decisions in life.

Acknowledgements are also in order to my *high school guidance counselor*, who told me when I was sixteen years old that I should give up my dream of becoming a physician, "because only two percent of medical students are women, and they got there because their fathers are doctors and their parents have money, neither of which is true in your case...besides which, I really don't think you're smart enough to be a doctor...so you probably shouldn't waste your time or your parents' hard-earned money on getting a college degree." (Thank goodness for my dad on that day, who told me: "Honey, if it's meant for you to be a doctor, there'll be a way."); and Kaye M. Coleman, PhD (1931-2015)—my *counselor* and co-founder of the Women's Resource Center at the University of Washington in early 1974—who contributed to my life in two significant ways. First, she helped me recognize that sleeping twelve hours per day and barely having enough energy to function at my job during the day for four months after my father unexpectedly died from a massive stroke two days after my twenty-sixth birthday was really *grief* and *not* depression. Second, she was the only person who looked at my work history, suggested career counseling in the form of three tests and, when she gave me the results, told me I was "smart enough to do just about anything you want to do." This was a big surprise to me, given my HS counselor's words ten years earlier! She then gave me *ten different professions* that I had scored almost equal interest in and aptitude for, one of which was medicine! At her suggestion and with her support, I took the entire next year to explore each and every one of them, at the end of which I chose medicine.

So, twenty years after *not* taking my HS guidance counselor's advice and after two other successful careers teaching and counseling, in addition to being only one course in statistics and a dissertation shy of a PhD in Health Services Administration, I entered osteopathic medical school. After graduating, I did an osteopathic rotating internship that steered me firmly in the direction of a more holistic family practice, including osteopathic manipulative medicine and acute homeopathy.

I started my private practice in Seattle at age forty-one...a life choice I have never regretted...because I felt like I had *finally* found my "calling" (life purpose). In honor of my maternal grandmother, Lillie Brown (whom I called Gram), who supported my dream of becoming a doctor for that entire twenty years, I opened my practice on her eighty-eighth birthday. She sent me a large, beautiful basket containing five plants, one of which was a small *Ficus benjamina* that lived for the first thirty years of my practice, and served as a constant reminder of the unconditional love and support I always felt from her. She "aged into health" until two months shy of her one-hundredth birthday. Dr. Gladys reminds me so much of her at times that I find myself paradoxically missing Gram more *and* less when I am with Dr. Gladys.

I also wish to express my deepest gratitude to the dedicated *teachers* I have been fortunate enough to have throughout my life, most especially:

My second grade teacher, for recognizing that my acting out and inattention in her class might be due to something more than purposeful misbehavior, and recommending that I be tested for "appropriate grade placement" (resulting in my being allowed to skip the third grade, *if* I could learn third grade math over the summer and pass a test on multiplication in the fall—which I did with the dedicated and loving help of my dad, who quit his very economically-needed second job to make that happen).

My fourth and fifth grade teacher, Mrs. Mincey, who correctly diagnosed my classroom misbehavior as boredom and whet my appetite for learning, inspiring me to want to follow in her footsteps and become a teacher myself someday, which then became my first career and part of every professional endeavor I have done since then.

Two outstanding professors from my days at BYU: Reed H. Bradford, PhD (1948-1994) who taught me the difference between religion and spirituality through the many intense conversations we had during his office hours and is only rivaled by Dr. Gladys in his ability to use real life situations to illustrate principles by telling a story, and Stephen R. Covey (1932-2012) who taught me principles that I live my life by to this day (*Spiritual Roots of Human Relations*, 1970; *The 7 Habits of Highly Effective People*, 1989; *Principle-Centered Leadership*, 1989; *First Things First*, 1994; *The 3rd Alternative*, 2011) and, together, are likely my equivalent influences as Dr. Gladys' Edgar Cayce (1877-1845).

Viola Frymann, DO (1921-2016) who taught me not only osteopathic manipulative therapy (OMT) skills, including cranial osteopathy—she deeply imprinted the *philosophy and principles* of osteopathy into my mind, heart, hands and soul—and left an indelible impression on me on the first day of medical school when she said to us: "If you do nothing else with your hands but treat newborn babies and resolve their birth trauma, you will have changed a child's life forever," which is very similar to Dr. Gladys' philosophy of the impact of giving *each* child a "loving birth."

Bernie Siegel, MD who shared with me the unique way that the Universe/God responds to his requests for guidance, which I still use to this day, and encouraged me to do an OMT-only family practice instead of surgery—"I'll save you ten years of your life, if you'll listen to me"—which I did and then taught a non-surgical, non-pharmacological approach to chronic pain nationally for five years with a holistic DDS and a podiatrist after receiving my first board certification in pain management in 1992.

Dietrich Klinghardt, MD/PhD and Louisa Williams, ND/DC who taught me the important contribution of the autonomic nervous system to enhance my ability to practice *individualized* holistic medicine, which I later termed *Non-protocol Medicine* (NPM), as Dr. Gladys had not yet come up with the term *Living Medicine*.

Devi Nambudripad, MD/PhD/DC/RN who taught me N.A.E.T. (Nambudripad's Allergy Elimination Technique) and led me to a deeper understanding of the work of Hans-Heinrich Recheweg, MD and homeopath (1905-1985) who "married" the principles of allopathic medicine and homeopathy, creating the field of homotoxicology to explain the mechanisms of chronic disease so that it can be treated *effectively*—principles that I still use in my practice to this day.

And last, though never least, Gladys Taylor McGarey, MD/MD (H)/ DABHM who has been my mentor for over thirty years now in both Holistic Medicine and Living Medicine, and without whose caring and support I would never have become the feisty female physician pioneer that I am under her tutelage. It was she who encouraged me to follow in her footsteps as the sole female physician with four male counterparts from the American Holistic Medical Association to champion the idea of a medical specialty board certification for holistic physicians through the creation and activation of the American Board of Holistic Medicine; and I did (1995-2000), from which over twenty-five thousand MD's and DO's became certified.

I will always be eternally grateful for those *patients/clients* in both my Washington and Arizona private practices who have allowed me to participate with them as their "Physician Without" in their healing process. In addition, I am likewise grateful for the populations of people I have *also* had the privilege of serving in southern Arizona that I was never exposed to in Washington: those with chronic pain who are opioid-addicted, those who are incarcerated, those with PTSD who have (at times) been suicidal, as well as veterans from all walks of life who rarely have access to more than a broken *disease*-care system.

While I do not have a study group like Dr. Gladys has to thank, I do want to acknowledge and express my deep appreciation for a handful of *close personal friends* who have supported me through thick and thin, who have loved me unconditionally, who *always* have my back and on whom I can absolutely count for honest feedback:

Ines Stolworthy Conover (1942-2019), whom I met at the age of nineteen, and was the first person who loved me *unconditionally* after I left home, to become a mutual and unwavering love between us for over fifty years.

Pat Speidel, one of my very first patients when I started my private practice in Seattle, has become a trusted colleague and friend through the years.

Arlene Sellereite, RN (retired) with whom I worked for almost thirteen years in my collaborative NPM practice (The Center for Optimal Health) and is still the reason I continue to travel to Seattle quarterly.

Jeanette Barrett who has been there for me in ways too numerous to mention, no matter how far apart we are in the world (she currently resides in Perth, Australia), including supporting me to stay on the planet when I thought my work here was done.

And Adam Huber, my soulmate in service to the world, who helps me remember the "big picture" of my life when I lose track of it and with whom I am writing the second edition of his book, *Red Toe Red Door[1]*, also soon to be published.

Lastly, I wish to acknowledge Donna Smith, a retired military veteran who served thirty-two years in the U.S. Army as a military intelligence all-source technician and was the first woman in that branch of service to achieve its highest rank of CW-5, for being the *initial* reason I ever considered leaving my beloved Northwest after nearly thirty years to come to Arizona; after which the Universe gave me

---

[1] www.metabolictherapy.org

fifteen other reasons! not the least of which was to reconnect with Dr. Gladys. Donna has been and continues to be a great support to me, both personally and professionally, for which I am very grateful.

Dedication

We dedicate this book to LIFE: the God-given Life Force which enlivens every molecule and every cell of our bodies.

We have watched with wonder as a pair of tiny glistening hummingbirds sit quietly for a while outside of Dr. Gladys' study and then speed off, as they continue their dance of life. As little as they are, and whether they know how beautiful they are or not, they bring love and healing to our souls. All parts of the Universe are interconnected and interdependent. Life and Love are the threads which hold it all together. Stephen Covey[2] perhaps best explains what we mean by this kind of interdependence that has allowed us to collaborate in such a joyful and effective way to achieve our goal (bold and italics are ours):

> **Interdependence** *is a far more mature, more advanced concept. If I am* **physically** *interdependent, I am self-reliant and capable, but I also realize that you and I working together can accomplish far more than, even at my best, I could accomplish alone. If I am* **emotionally** *interdependent, I de-rive a great sense of worth within myself, but I also recognize the need for love, for giving and for receiving love from others. If I am* **intellectually** *interdependent, I realize that I need the best thinking of other people to join with my own.*

---

[2] Covey, Stephen. *The 7 Habits of Highly Effective People*, 1989.

Foreword

When I ponder the fact that Dr. Gladys was the same age when she became my mentor that I was when I came to Arizona in 2017, I am truly humbled by the synchronicity of Life. Coming to a state in which I had done six months of clinical rotations in 1985-86 and swore never to return to has truly made me eat my words. No matter how many times Dr. Gladys and I saw each other or spoke on the phone in the years before 2017, I never said yes to her invitations to join her in practice in Arizona. However, now that I have been here for a little over three years, spending much of my time working closely with her, both personally and professionally, I have learned to appreciate the desert climate that Dr. Gladys so loves and the rural lifestyle in which I now find myself living. Both have grown on me...as has she.

    I can also tell you that Dr. Gladys and I have *both* grown in extraordinary ways during this writing process. The following image is the best way for me to illustrate this point, explain this experience and demonstrate one way of understanding Living Medicine. It is also the logo[3] I have used in my practice since 1994 to explain to my patients how we will work *together* during their healing journey.

---

[3] ©1995 by Ann Brown McCombs, DO.

This is an artist's rendition of the Auguste Rodin sculpture of two right hands that I have had in my office for over twenty-five years (in this rendition, it is two *left* hands). The hands represent two people working *equally* together (not in a one-up/one-down power differential way), in the presence of the Life Force (the golden-orange energy *between* their hands), to come up with a *unique* solution to whatever problem (or issue) they are trying to solve (or resolve), which I have always called the *Divine 3rd Alternative* (represented by the white light of the diamond or crystal between them coming down from the heavens or Collective Unconscious).

This metaphor represents the essence of the experience Dr. Gladys and I had while writing this book, and the metaphor is applicable throughout it. For example, the two hands could represent the science and art of medicine, conventional and holistic medicine, the Physician Within and the Physician Without, Life and Love, etc. The white light would then represent the *unique* ways Living Medicine can be applied to blend these concepts in the first three examples and the Divine Spark that ignites Life and Love in the last example. What I can say, in working with Dr. Gladys in this way, is that the challenge was always to listen to her words (often channeled, in my opinion, from some other dimension) and translate them into two-dimensional language in *her own* voice. After many edits of this book *together*, we both believe that we have done that...and feel grateful and humbled by the process.

Being with Dr. Gladys while writing this second edition of her signature work has also given me the opportunity to *fully* appreciate the kind of practice I have been fortunate enough to have for more than thirty-one years now: "non-managed" care, non-insurance-based, focused on *healing* from the *root causes* of illness and managing symptom treatment using pharmaceuticals and surgery as a *last* resort...all of the things Dr. Gladys writes about in this edition of her book. I have both her and Andrew Taylor Still, DO (the founder of osteopathy) to thank for that opportunity.

No matter how full my day is or how challenging the patients are that I see, I almost always feel better at the *end* of my day than I did at the beginning. Many patients and physicians with whom I come in contact report their daily experiences to be just the opposite. I trust both will be inspired, as I continue to be, by Dr. Gladys' words and the stories (*all of which are true*) that she has chosen to share in this edition. As I learned from my dear professor of sociology at BYU and continue to learn from Dr. Gladys: "ideas are remembered best when punctuated by **a good story**."[4] These two great storytellers in the modern world both rival Jesus' skill in using parables **to teach** these **important ideas**, which we have **called principles**. (In this edition, you cannot miss them: the principles are all in BOLD!) As I learned early on from Stephen Covey[5] (bold, non-italics are mine):

> As a **principle-centered person**, *you **see** things differently. And because you see things differently, you **think** differently, you **act** differently.* [And] *because you have a high degree of security, guidance, wisdom and power that flows from a solid, unchanging core, you* [not only] *have the foundation of a highly proactive and...effective life...*[you have the foundation for making a shift into the Living Medicine paradigm. In that paradigm, we] *are free to choose our actions, based on our knowledge of **correct** principles, but we are not free to choose the consequences of those actions. Remember, "if you pick up one end of the stick, you pick up the other."*

In choosing to do a few short-term *locum tenens* assignments in between writing times with Dr. Gladys—all of which were in "managed

---

[4] Bradford, Reed, PhD. *And They Shall Teach Their Children*, 1965.

[5] Covey, Stephen. *The 7 Habits of Highly Effective People*, 1989.

care" environments in southern Arizona —I can now understand how some doctors become disillusioned, even "burned- out," while working in that kind of environment and sometimes feel like they are selling their souls for money. I also observed that the patients in those settings rarely felt important, much less cared for.

Following those experiences, I made two promises to myself: First, to do everything in my power to *never* have to work in that kind of environment *ever again*; and, secondly, to commit to finding another way to work in these wisdom years of my life to fulfill my life purpose of being a physician who lives with integrity and makes a significant difference in the lives of others. Dr. Gladys has been and continues to be my inspiration for these commitments. I can honestly say that happiness turns into joy for me *every time* we are together, and it has been especially so in our collaboration to transform this second edition of *Living Medicine* into a textbook to teach these principles and concepts to both physicians *and* patients.

Out of this book, our hope is that physicians will be able to become the physicians *they* want to be…patients will learn how to connect with *their* Physician Within, as well how to find the Physicians Without that *they* want to work with…and *both* will see that they each have a *choice* to settle for nothing less. **Living Medicine is the paradigm shift that is needed *now* for medicine to be able to heal *itself***, so that patients *and* physicians can feel safe, protected and secure enough to do the deep healing work that they *both* need to do to bring about *true* healing.

Thank you, Mother/Father/God/Universe for Dr. Gladys Taylor McGarey and for this amazing opportunity to give back to this extraordinary woman for all she has done for me and continues to do for herself, her profession and the world. She is known as (and has been affectionately called) the "Mother of Holistic Medicine." I think she has now lived long enough to see her progeny grow and expand in this field to have earned two *new* titles: the "*Grandmother* of Holistic Medicine" and now the "*Mother* of Living Medicine." I am doing, and will continue to do, all I can to assist The Foundation for Living Medicine to complete Dr. Gladys' Legacy Project during her lifetime, the first of which is this second edition of her signature work, as well as assist in the creation and implementation of her ultimate vision, the Village for Living Medicine.

Please join me on this journey of recognizing, appreciating and memorializing one of the *truly great* medical pioneers of our time...an icon, for sure...and one who *also* has her feet of clay planted firmly on the ground, "walking her talk" to the best of her ability, in *every* moment of *every* day. I know this because I have worked, eaten and slept in *her* home of Living Medicine, up close and personal. I have treated her, cooked for her, loved her and cared for her. I treasure every conversation we have ever had, intense or mundane. Why? Because Dr. Gladys *lives* life, *loves* life and *labors* to incorporate these **Living Medicine principles** into her life 24/7, *laughing* as she turns lemons into lemonade, always *listening* for that "still small voice" to guide her and teach her, with every breath and step she takes (her goal is three thousand per day!). It is an honor to be her witness as well as her translator, occasional spokesperson and frequent chauffeur. Enjoy the ride...she certainly does!

Ann B. McCombs, DO, DABHM, DNM
Sierra Vista, Arizona

Summer, 2020

Preface to the Second Edition

I have worked my whole life as a physician with a primary focus on healing. The fact that medicine has changed throughout my many years in practice, along with my perception of the work of my colleagues whose healing practices focus on *energy medicine*, inspired me to write the second edition of this book.

I felt called to make note of the changes I have both observed and experienced since writing the first edition and bring them to the attention of myself, first of all, and then to all who work in the field of medicine—and, in fact, to *anyone* who accepts that **the "Physician Within" is a *living* entity.**

This idea has been known since the time of Hippocrates, who said: "If you are not your own doctor, you are a fool."[6] That awareness precipitated an "aha" moment for me when I realized that *true* **healing cannot come about until a person learns to work with the Physician Within** *as well as* **the Physician Without.** So, when people ask me what kind of audience I wrote this book for, my response is: "for people," because *each one of us* has our own Physician Within (our intuitive part) that has to learn to work with a Physician Without (the physician or any other health care provider that we have chosen to work with) whenever we are challenged with a health problem to solve. Thus, both physicians *and* patients can benefit from this second edition, I believe, even though I am primarily writing it from my point of view as a physician.

---

[8] https://quotefancy.com>quote>Hippocrates.

For *true* healing to happen, we must learn what it feels like to see things from another person's point of view, i.e. "walk a mile in [another's] shoes"[7] or "climb into [another's] skin and walk around in it,"[8] because **healing is a two-way street**. So, in short, even though you will find that I am often directing my comments to physicians, I am actually speaking to *everyone* who reads this book.

As a small child, I grew up in India watching my parents work with the people in the villages of northern India. My parents were both osteopathic (DO) physicians serving as medical missionaries. My dad also earned his MD degree by completing an ophthalmology residency in 1912. (His book about their time there is now in the process of being reprinted: see below.) I knew that their concern for people's welfare as *total* beings—body, mind and spirit —was essential to their work.

I knew that the diseases the Indian people contracted and the physical traumas they were living through were all part of their *total* life experiences and that the purpose of my parents' work was to help them LIVE their lives as fully as possible, instead of just focusing on their diseases. Sometimes, they were able to ease their patients' pain. Sometimes, they were able to give them medication that allowed them to survive a bout of malaria. Sometimes, they were able to help with the birth of a baby and, sometimes, it was just pulling a painful tooth. I knew they served in the villages as *agents of love*, caring for and offering hope to their patients.

As medical missionaries, my parents were paid by the church that had sent them to India, so there was never an exchange of money. Occasionally, one of the people would bring a gift. However, the service rendered was just that—*service*, given freely—from the grateful hearts of my physician parents. As I thought about becoming a doctor, the idea that the practice of medicine would, out of necessity, become a business with an exchange of money seemed foreign to me. I had to learn that paying for a doctor's visit was essential to the practice of

[7] www.grammarist.com>phrase>walk>a>mile>in>someone>else's>shoes.

[8] Finch, Atticus to Scout in To Kill A Mockingbird, 1960.

medicine, although I never really understood this necessary component. It was almost as if the financial part of the practice of medicine
was an "add-on" and not really at the *heart* of the work that I felt called
to do.

How many other physicians have felt this way as they went into
medicine? I do not know. I would not be surprised, however, since
medicine *has* become a major business—to practice it, physicians
must now think of it that way—and is something that many physicians-
in-training haven't anticipated or, on a deeper level, really understand.
Be that as it may, the fact remains that the practice of medicine *is* a
business and, to survive in this field, physicians have had to learn
about this business.

The term *conventional medicine* is used to identify the allopathic
approach to healing that has been taught in medical and osteopathic schools since the Flexner Report (a book-length study of medical education in the U.S. and Canada written by Abraham Flexner)
was published in 1910 under the aegis of the Carnegie Foundation.[9]
It is what most MD's practice. "The term 'allopathy' was coined in
1810 by Samuel Hahnemann, MD (1755-1843) to designate the usual
practice of medicine [using drugs and surgery to treat disease] as
opposed to *homeopathy*, the system of therapy that he founded [in
1796[10]]. Allopathic medicine refers broadly to medical practice that is
also termed Western medicine, evidence-based medicine or modern
medicine. Homeopathy is based on the concept that disease can be
treated with minute doses of drugs [remember that plants were the
original source of many pharmaceuticals that were later synthesized
in the laboratory] thought capable of producing the same symptoms
in healthy people as the disease itself."[11]

*Philosophically, these two approaches are diametrically opposite
in the way they approach the treatment of disease.* "Allopathic medi-

[9] www.ScienceDirect.com>topics>flexner-report.

[10] www.ncbi.nlm.nih.gov>pmc1676328.

[11] Shiel, William C. Jr, MD. "Medical Definition of Allopathic Medicine" (reviewed
12/21/18), www.medicinenet.com.

cines attempt to alleviate the symptoms of disease by attacking/affecting the natural defense of the body, whereas homeopathy embraces the body's natural response system by treating either the symptoms of healing or attacking the root cause of the illness."[12] Dr. Ann highly recommends the books by Harris L. Coulter, PhD[13] (1932-2009) for anyone interested in understanding *the history of Western medical philosophy* from the time of Hippocrates to the twentieth century *as a unified system of thought* versus "a series of fortuitous discoveries." As the leading medical historian of the twentieth century, Dr. Ann thinks Dr. Coulter's books should be *required reading* for *every* medical student. She knows of no better way for students to gain both a "big picture" overview as well as an appreciation for the *roots* of their chosen profession.

The conventional approach to medicine has led to magnificent strides in the *science* of medicine, involving medications, therapeutic procedures and amazing surgical advances. Untold numbers of lives have been saved with this approach to medicine. The quality of conventional medicine, which deals primarily with *disease*, is unsurpassed. However, it is still very apparent to me that, **with conventional medicine, a physician may cure the disease and still not heal the patient.** Conversely, I have also seen patients heal whose disease was not cured! Nevertheless, *the primary focus of modern medicine,* no matter what term is used to describe it (or what modality is used to practice it) *still centers on eradicating disease and disease processes.* In so doing, **conventional medicine has taken the power away from the *living* process and given it instead to the *disease* process, which operates within a context of *killing* instead of *healing.***

For many years I have attempted to balance the current reality of the *practice* of conventional medicine with what I know is my *true*

---

[12] Sultan, A. et.al. "Allopathy versus Homeopathy: A Never Ending Tacit War," Medicinal Chemistry , Volume 6(4): 239-240 (2016), www.hilarispublisher.com.

[13] Coulter, Harris L. PhD. Divided Legacy (Volumes I-IV) – published originally in 1975, 1977, 1993, 1994.

"calling." First and foremost, I consider myself a partner to the *healing* process, so the direction my profession has taken concerns me. Like my parents, I believe that to have *true* healing, physicians must not only look at the body and disease; we must also treat people as *total* beings—body, mind *and* spirit—as well as help them reclaim a reverence for Life...whether in birthing, dying or anywhere in between. It was out of my concern about this issue that the concept of Living Medicine emerged for me one day when I was talking to friends. I made the statement that medicine, as it is *currently* being practiced, represents a "killing machine" that needs to change its focus from killing to *living*. I then stopped, raised my arms to the heavens, and said: "Thank you! I have been waiting many years for that term!" (Living Medicine).

As the concept of Living Medicine began to emerge for me, I also realized that—in the process of bringing back into the practice of medicine the *heart* of medicine—the energy of the Feminine must be *re*-incorporated *along with* **the *art* of medicine**, as it **is just as important as the *science* of medicine**. I also realized that, **until physicians focus on Life and living, they are not dealing *realistically* with the human condition**—nor can they be as helpful in the healing process—and *true* healing cannot take place. This principle also holds true for all those in need of healing: **if patients hand over the responsibility for their healing process *completely* to their physician or any other health care provider, they are diminishing their *own* power in the healing process**.

Over the years that I have lived with these emerging concepts, the following **basic tenets of Living Medicine** have evolved:

1. Living Medicine is Life itself...and Life itself *is* Living Medicine.
2. Living Medicine becomes the reality when we can tune in to our *own* life to such an extent that *living* it becomes the healer.
3. Life itself creates the medicine we need for healing. This requires "at-one-ment" with the Physician Within and cooperation with the Physician Without.

4. Our challenge in Living Medicine is to access the Life Force. This requires being present in *every* moment of our life so that, if circumstances present us with illness or catastrophe *or* joy and laughter, we can use *all* of it to enhance and support that Life Force.

Because Living Medicine teaches that Life itself is the healer, **our focus as Living Medicine physicians must *always* be on supporting and enhancing the Life Force.** Sometimes this means dealing with a disease or getting rid of an aspect of our life (or even a body part) that no longer enhances Life itself, which could involve *any* aspect of allopathic medicine *or* be as simple as getting a haircut! From the Living Medicine perspective, the *primary* focus would be on Life and Living *instead of* just striving to eliminate diseases. **Any therapeutic intervention or modality that enhances the Life Force is part of Living Medicine.** For example, homeopathy *focuses* on enhancing the Life Force. Color, music, acupuncture, nutrition, massage and dance all *enhance* the Life Force and can thus also be parts of Living Medicine. There can even be times that allopathic medicines and procedures (including surgery) play this role. **Love, joy and balance are the very heart of Living Medicine, which is healing from the inside out *instead of* from the outside in.** While it is important for physicians to know and incorporate these Living Medicine principles in the healing process, **it is *equally* important that patients know these principles also, and then hold their doctors to this standard.** With physicians and patients working *together* in this way, the foundation for *true* healing can be laid, and the *best* chance for *deep* healing becomes possible. It is also the best way to turn off any and all *external* voices suggesting that we are *victims* of our disease process, and/or that it is impossible to heal from *any* disease, much less learn to *live* with it peacefully and joyfully.

I have lived in the arena of modern medicine since the day I was born, having come into this life knowing the medical profession was my path. My physician mother went into labor with me at her first sight of the Taj Mahal, the magnificent tomb of Mumtaz Mahal, which I believe is a temple built to honor the Divine Feminine in labor. I have written the second edition of this book with the hope that the concept of Living Medicine will help physicians to merge *all* the realities that are manifesting in the practice of medicine at the present time and make it a "win-win" or good situation for all concerned. I also hope that the medical profession can incorporate healing on the *monetary* level as well as holistically, since we live in a world where finances must be looked at, because they are part of the physical dimension in which we live. In addition, I have written this second edition as a physician who recognizes the Physician Within *each person* will be reading this revised and updated book, and, as practicing physicians, we frequently find ourselves *also* in the role of patient. My hope is that the role of the Physician Within *each person* will become recognized, so that the Physician *Within* can learn to communicate clearly and effectively with the Physician *Without*, no matter which role we find ourselves in.

I have also written a myriad of articles and spoken on numerous subjects related to the field of medicine for many years. Although the things I wrote and said in the 1960's are inherently the same today, Life and Living have added dimensions of understanding and a deep-ened awareness of the fundamental nature of medicine. Stories have grown up around my work in such a way that my practice of medicine *evolved* into a Living Medicine practice, where *true* healing became a *living* process that focused on Life and growth instead of death and killing. Now, in my one-hundredth year, my deepest desire is to leave a legacy that will assist practicing physicians and other health care professionals, as well as physicians-in-training, to become *whole* physicians and health care providers. I believe that when caregivers are given the opportunity to experience *true* healing as part of *their* personal and professional lives, they can then assist their patients to do the same. I also hope that my legacy will cement the understanding of and an appreciation for the fact that **all of us have within *each* of us our own Physician Within.** It is that part of us that carries the *individual* and *personal* wisdom about the kind of medicine that con-tributes *best* to assist *each one of us* on our very individual and deeply personal healing journey.

On the Fourth of July in 1993, I moved into my new little house that was built in my daughter (Helene)'s backyard. Since then, it has become my home and my dwelling place. It has also become a meta-phor for my concept of Living Medicine. Although I had not planned for Independence Day to be my move-in day, it became a metaphor for gathering my independent thoughts about medicine. Since I have lived with the practice of medicine for almost a hundred years now, *it also* has become my home and my dwelling place. Using my home as a metaphor provides an opportunity to share my ideas and concepts about this great profession that has been a part of my life for so many years.

So, come with me now as I retrace my steps in building *my* Liv-ing Medicine home. My prayer is that you will take these ideas and concepts and build *your own* home of Living Medicine, so that it be-comes *your own* personal dwelling place as well…the place where *your* body, mind and spirit can blossom, grow and mature…evolving *your* being—slowly, but surely—day by day—into the valuable, con-tributing member of the *truly* human race that you were destined to become. This is the ideal I actively strive to achieve through the per-sonal and professional choices I make in *every* moment of *every* day. Please join me on this incredible journey to wholeness, peace and love. I welcome you with open arms!

Gladys T. McGarey, MD, MD (H), DABHM
Scottsdale, Arizona
Summer, 2020

Chapter Overviews

Chapter One: The Groundbreaking

This chapter introduces the metaphor of a home to describe the *conventional* practice of medicine and how it compares with *osteopathic* medicine. It identifies the place where we can look at concepts and practices in the field of medicine as the ground on which we will build our home/practice of Living Medicine. Some of these concepts do *not* contribute to Life and healing (e.g. treating the symptoms vs. the causes of disease states, losing track of the *patient* in our search for identifying and treating these disease states and/or insisting on prolonging a person's life when it is *their* choice not to do so), and need to be either removed or reviewed and clarified from a Living Medicine perspective. These concepts are important to include, however, to help us better understand—in the *context* of Living Medicine—how they apply to *all* of us (physicians and patients alike), as *there will never be a time when physicians will not be in the patient role at some point in their life.*

Chapter Two: The Foundation

In this chapter we see that for the foundation of Living Medicine to be solid and stable, it needs to have the proper mix of the art (spirit) *and* science (mind) of medicine in order to work effectively to heal the physical form (body) manifesting *any* disease state. In Living Medicine, the physician is seen not only as the doctor, s/he is also recognized as the patient. **The physician-patient relationship is *primary* in the Living Medicine paradigm, and it is held as sacrosanct.**

The Life Force, as manifested in the *chakra* system (the major energy centers of the body), is properly placed in the foundation. Our emotions are controlled by these energy centers, which manifest in each of the physical body's endocrine glands. A solid *and* stable foundation in this paradigm also requires that *all* aspects of the body be integrated and work well together for *true* healing and *optimal* health to have a real chance of happening. The concept of *tensegrity* is discussed as one way this foundation can be created to manifest these outcomes, using OMT and the physician-dentist team as examples of this important principle.

Chapter Three: The Living Room
In Living Medicine, this room is the metaphor we use to understand how we allow situations and emotions to enter our physical environment. In this chapter, we identify who we are, how we want to be seen in the world *and* how to care for *ourselves*. How emotions affect us physically, mentally, emotionally and spiritually is also addressed in this chapter, as well as the principle that **Life is both the Great Teacher *and* the Great Healer in the Living Medicine paradigm.**

Chapter Four: The Kitchen and Dining Room
The food we eat is not just for the nourishment of our *physical* body. *What we feed our mind and spirit is just as important.* *How* our food is prepared, as well as how we *feel* when preparing it, affects not only *our* total being, it also impacts the body, mind and spirit of the people for whom we prepare it. This effect is reflected in the way the food is presented. All these principles determine how well we are *ultimately* nourished by the food we eat. In this chapter, we learn that emotions also affect how our body *uses* the food we eat, and that **we must first learn how to *truly* nourish *ourselves* before we can nourish others *effectively*.**

Chapter Five: The Library
The library chapter is a metaphor to examine the *history of medicine* as well as *my own* personal and professional journey as a physi-

cian. My 80-year journey (to date!) has involved learning *conventional* medicine, pioneering the emergence of *holistic medicine* and now reinventing the practice of medicine yet again in my one-hundredth year by evolving *Living Medicine.* To embrace this next paradigm shift in the field of medicine, I had to grasp the concept that **I had to** *first* **understand what I had been taught** *before* **I could learn what I needed to learn.** In my journey as a physician, I very quickly saw that *it was* not enough *to just learn skills and modalities,* conventional or holistic. I discovered that I had to *use* those skills and modalities to understand Life and Living in order to do *more than* just treat my patients' symptoms, *if* I wanted to bring about *true* healing. My journey included learning the *Edgar Cayce material,*[14] which I found very helpful in so many ways in my efforts to understand and appreciate the growth of the concept of the *Feminine* Face of medicine. These two concepts are introduced in this chapter, followed by many examples of how they both relate to and impact Living Medicine.

Chapter Six: The Bedroom

The bedroom chapter is a metaphor to understand **the importance of having the conscious** *and* **unconscious minds meet each other.** Where this meeting occurs is *not* about a specific location, as this meeting place is unique to *each* person. Finding this healing place for *ourselves,* though, is what will foster the discovery of how *our own* conscious and unconscious minds intersect and interact with each other. It then becomes the place where we can experience and understand birth and death, rest and healing, as well as the importance of our *dreams* and the insights provided by meditation. Last, though certainly not least, this healing place also provides a personal space for love and growth.

---

[14] www.edgarcayce.org and www.encyclopedia.com>science>contemporary>mystery >schools>and>reincarnation. This May 31, 2020 update specifically quotes Dr. Gladys regarding how her understanding of the Cayce material influences her practice of medicine. It also explains where Edgar Cayce fits in the history of these modern mystery schools.

Chapter Seven: The Playroom

The playroom chapter is the metaphor employed to learn **the importance of *balancing* work and play**, and that there is truth in the old saying that "all work and no play makes Jack (or Jill) a dull boy (or girl)." *One person's work may be another person's play.* Gaining the understanding that learning to balance these two important aspects of our lives is the *only* way to achieve a *truly* abundant life on *every* level. In addition, as we learn to stretch and grow beyond our *perceived* limits, risk-taking on *all* levels may be required.

Chapter Eight: The Bathroom

In this chapter, the bathroom is the metaphor used to teach the importance of **learning to deal *effectively* with assimilation and elimination on *all* levels of our being—body, mind and spirit**. In this chapter, we discuss that detoxification is necessary on *all* these levels, as well as the specific ways that it can be accomplished physically, emotionally, mentally and spiritually.

Chapter Nine: The Garden

This chapter is the metaphor for learning that the garden is more than the front and back yards of our home. It **represents the *conscious* face we present to the world (front yard) as well as the work that goes on in our *unconscious* (backyard)**. Not only is our garden a *physical* place where we can learn to interact with Mother Nature and our environment in a *responsible* way (including caring for Mother Earth), it is also the emotional, mental and spiritual place where we can learn to interact with ourselves and others (colleagues, staff, patients, friends, partners and families in *all* forms) in gentle, yet effective, ways.

Chapter Ten: The Back Porch

This chapter is a metaphor to emphasize the importance of learning to see the "big picture" in all situations as well as the importance of learning the skill of effective self-reflection. The value of watching sunsets helps us see the importance of what we have accomplished thus far in our lives. This chapter also discusses the value of learning to "think outside-the-box" in medicine. In so doing, **physicians learn to value their contributions to the *future* of medicine, as well as assess their ability to effectively examine the *roots* of its past.** When patients learn to think in this way also, they can better hear their Physician Within. They can then become an *even better* partner with their Physician Without, as they journey *together* in the healing process. To reach the solution that serves the Highest Good of *all* concerned, we summarize the principles that will lead us to the paradigm shift that *must* happen to support the field of medicine and transform its broken "disease care" system back into the health care system it was always meant to be: *Living* Medicine.

1

The Groundbreaking

A house remains a house until Life has been brought into it. Then it becomes a home. When we start to build a home, we need an architect to help with the plans and to create a blueprint. When the blueprint is in hand, we begin the work of manifesting these concepts on the earth in a two-dimensional way, because *everything* on the earth exists within the consciousness of "duality" (sperm and ovum, male and female, light and dark, positive and negative, good and evil, right and wrong, etc.). In building a house, we must start the construction by digging into and moving the earth. Likewise, in preparing for the construction of our home of Living Medicine, we will have to deepen the way we think about Life and healing.

In our house of Living Medicine, there are some teachings we learned in medical school that were touted to be the truth. While today I find some of these facts no longer useful, they are still in the earth on which our house of Living Medicine is being built. Some of these things can be easily shifted and moved. Others are like coming upon a great rock that needs to be completely removed or broken apart. One of these rocks is that **the practice of medicine represents a war against disease.** This huge rock labeled "Attack and Destroy the Disease" cannot just be hauled away. It must be broken down and repositioned. Although diseases will continue to present the issues that Living Medicine will deal with, they can now be identified as *opportunities* (instead of enemies) to access *true* healing. **While the** individual disease processes underlie the entire structure of our home of Living Medicine, they do not represent the *primary* soil upon which the structure is built. We may need to break down and redistribute the ground our Living Medicine home is built upon so that, if a disease occurs, it can find its *proper* place. *Our* focus is going to be on building a *living* structure that will incorporate the presence of the disease and make it part of the *useful* energy upon which we build...just as, in the martial arts, the *chi* energy that comes toward us is *not* obstructed or destroyed, but is used instead to further the action intended for the practice of this sport. The energy of healing is likewise used in a constructive way to enhance the Life Force.

The medicine I was taught in medical school (which is still generally practiced today) is not *just* a war against disease—IT IS A KILLING MACHINE. We *kill* bacteria, *eradicate* AIDS, *eliminate* diabetes and so forth. *When our whole focus is on death, not Life, we cannot live Life to its fullest.* Even our everyday language itself does *not* affirm Life. We talk about *anti*biotics, *anti*depressants, *ant*acids and even *anti*-aging. (As a newly-minted centenarian, that one really gets me!) Women talk about *fighting* osteoporosis as if they want to destroy their own bones. If the focus of our work as doctors is primarily to *destroy* the disease process, then we need more and more ammunition with which to do this—which, of course, includes many kinds of medications and often invasive procedures, surgery being the main one.

In 1955 the *Physician's Desk Reference* was half-an-inch thick. Now it is at least *three* inches thick with three addenda...or we can now just look it up on a PDR "app" or Google! The more we find ammunition to kill "the disease," the more that ammunition itself can and does create *iatrogenic* (any unintended event resulting from medical treatment) problems that have no end, just as the whole concept of war has no end. Bacteria are constantly becoming resistant to antibiotics, with no end to this process in sight. Viruses have become epidemic, and some even pandemic during my lifetime (e.g. the Spanish flu of 1918 and now COVID-19 in 2020). World War I was supposed to be the war to end all wars. Maybe **it is time we started to think about addressing the disease process from a different angle.** If patients are also considered to be *spiritual* beings, then each patient has a destiny with spiritual influences that can and often do have a direct bearing on their health. This paradigm would mean that we should **approach the patient as a *whole* person and not just as a disease diagnosis.** Our job then becomes about **bringing healing to the *person* vs. simply curing, alleviating or destroying a *disease*.** Because an individual has a purpose for living, **the person's *whole* being**—including his or her past work, emotions and thoughts—**plays a part in the illness that s/he is currently manifesting.** This concept *will require a shift in approach for most physicians who have been allopathically trained*, as well as for individuals who have only experienced being a patient in that paradigm. *It will also require setting an example.* For physicians who have been *osteopathically* trained, however, these Living Medicine concepts fit like a hand in a glove! This is because, as a distinct branch of medicine in the U.S., **osteopathic medicine** *emphasizes the interrelated unity of all systems, each working with the other to heal the* whole *body* in times of illness.[15] As fully-licensed physicians in all fifty states, DO's practice their unique **whole-person approach** in every medical specialty as well. This philosophical difference is in addition to the fact that all DO's complete *additional training in osteopathic manipulative therapy* (OMT), a hands-on tool to assist with diagnosing, treating and preventing injury and illness. As a result, DO's take a seventh National Board Exam in addition to the six that all MD's and DO's take (three in basic science and three in clinical medicine). *Both professions* practice medicine according to the latest science and technology, and they can cross-train at the graduate (residency) level in *any* medical specialty they choose. DO's, however, also consider *options in addition to drugs and surgery*, using those allopathic tools as a *last* resort instead of first-response therapy. Because both of my parents were DO's, this philosophy and style of practicing medicine was a part

---

[15] www.osteopathic.org>AmericanOsteopathicAssociation>what-is-osteopathic-medicine

of my life from the time I was born. Dr. Ann was fortunate enough to have been treated by a DO at the age of fourteen, even though it took her another twenty-two years to find her way into this profession. I can personally attest to her skills in this arena, and I love the handouts[16] she originated for her patients to illustrate and explain the differences between these two types of medicine.

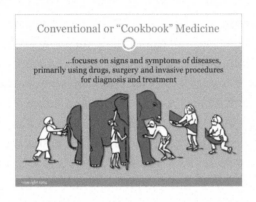

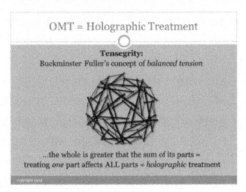

I graduated from medical school in 1946 just as World War II had ended and received my training in medicine during the entire length of the war. I started as a freshman at Women's Medical College in Philadelphia in September 1941, and the war started on December 7th of that same year. Antibiotics were discovered during this time, and sulfa

---

[16] McCombs, Ann, DO. Text written by Dr. Ann and original artwork commissioned by her, ©1994.

and penicillin became lifesaving agents. Amazing surgical procedures were developed and perfected, and our ability to repair the damages that were done to the human body during this time was quite awe-inspiring. We also began to understand a little bit about what war does to the *mind* of a human being and the damage that can occur to a person's psyche as a result of it (referred to as "soldier's heart" during the Civil War, "shell shock"—a term coined by Charles Myers[17]—after WW I, "battle fatigue" or Combat Stress Reaction/CSR after WW II[18] and now known as "post-traumatic stress disorder"/PTSD). The war was all around us. The news was full of it; the medical profession was perfecting skills to deal with it; and I had classmates whose husbands were in Guam and Europe. Bill McGarey and I were married in 1943 when he was in the V-12 program, preparing to be a physician in the Navy. Throughout those four years, there was never a moment that war was not part of our living, breathing life. Food products were rationed, gas was rationed, tires were rationed. Every tire you put on your car was one that was recapped, because you could not buy new ones. Medical supplies were scarce. We did not complain, however: we were "at war."

After WW II, our attitude toward disease in the medical profession did not change. Disease was still our enemy and, as physicians, we were taught to identify and destroy it. **The concept that the purpose of the practice of medicine is to get rid of disease has not changed through the years; it has only become *more* ingrained and sophisticated.** Patients think that this purpose is what physicians are to do for them; and we, as physicians, are constantly under the gun to learn new ways to accomplish this goal. Dr. Ann pointed out to me that Dr. Coulter[19] understood this fact "in spades," referring to this concept as the "*medical monopoly*":

---

[17] Butterworth, BR. "What World War I taught us about PTSD" (Nov 8, 2018), www.theconversation.com.

[18] Friedman, MD/PhD, MJ. "History of PTSD in Veterans: Civil War to DSM-5" (Oct 17, 2019), www.ptsd.va.gov.

[19] Coulter, Harris L. PhD. Divided Legacy (Volume III), 1993.

> *Society today is paying a heavy price in disease and death for the monopoly granted the medical profession in the 1920's* [when the Flexner Report was fully implemented in medical education]. *In fact, the situation peculiarly resembles that of the 1830's when physicians relied on bloodletting, mercurial medicines and quinine... knowing them to be intrinsically harmful. And precisely the same arguments were made in defense of these medicines as are employed today, namely that the benefits outweigh the risks. In truth, the benefits accrue to the physicians, while the patient runs the risks.*

We both agree with Dr. Coulter's assessment, though we would probably change his term for this concept to the "*allopathic* monopoly" to be fair to osteopathic medicine (developed in 1874 by Andrew Taylor Still, MD), as well as the other forms of medicine that originated both *before* (e.g. Chinese medicine, Ayurvedic medicine and homeopathy, to name just a few) and *after* (e.g. holistic medicine, Living Medicine) allopathic medicine was distinguished and defined by Dr. Hahnemann in 1810. We also find it interesting that all forms of medicine *other than allopathic* are termed "CAM" (complementary and alternative medicine), all of which are discussed in detail in Chapter 2. The impact of this monopoly on physicians, however—no matter what term is used to describe it —is significant, as the following story illustrates.

In the mid-1970's, I was waiting for an obstetrical patient of mine to birth her baby at Doctor's Hospital in Phoenix. It was about three o'clock in the morning, and a friend of mine (another family physician, Jack McCarville, MD (1926-2016) was also waiting for his patient to give birth. We talked a lot about conditions in the medical profession that night. He commented: "The problem with medicine now is that the fun has all gone out of it." I pondered his statement for many years, and *still* wonder about it, because I really wasn't sure at the time what he was talking about. I think I now know. By "fun" he didn't mean laughter and play—he meant the real *joy* that we felt when we were working with people and contacting the very essence of who they are and what we could do to help them. It was why we both went into medicine to begin with: To become a part of **the doctor/patient relationship**, the essence of which **is the excitement that goes along with watching patients contact that *inner* aspect of themselves and, as a result, manifest the magnificence of their human spirit.** Often, in the direst of circumstances, it is the awareness that **our support of the patient**, whether it is through medication or surgery or any other modality, **is vital to the healing process** and, therefore, creates a bond between us and the patient that is *truly* an aspect of love in its purest form. I call this process **contacting the Physician Within** a patient.

In Donna Zajonc's book, *The Politics of Hope,*[20] she discusses some concepts that I feel relate very closely to Living Medicine. She says: "As leaders, we consistently move our focus away from problem solving *per se* and focus on how to sustain a balanced life for all of the world's inhabitants." As I look at that statement and put it in context with my thoughts about Living Medicine, I believe this: **as long as we are concentrating on the disease and the destruction of the disease, we do not have the energy *or* the focus to work with the Life Force itself, because Life itself is the Great Healer, and the *only* thing that can bring about *true* healing.**

Zajonc says: "When we focus on problems, our energy is directed toward what we *don't* want [the problems] rather than what we *do* want. Our vision, like our goal, is limited to getting rid of the irritant, rather than focusing on creating something delightfully effective or even artful. **The more energy we place on solving problems, the more [those] problems in general will [affect] our lives.** [The aspects of whatever problem we are trying to solve] begin to define ev-

[20] Zajonc, Donna. *The Politics of Hope: Reviving the Dream of Democracy – A Guide to Political Renewal for Our Times,* 2004.

ery conversation. It's an insidious trap, but the problem focus keeps us mentally confined to very close quarters." We could change the word "problems" to *diseases* and say: *"When we focus on diseases, our energy is directed toward what we do* not *want—the diseases— rather than what we* do *want—healing."*

This concept can be compared to the forming of a pearl. The oyster finds a grain of sand in its shell and begins to incorporate that grain of sand into its very essence, so that the sand is no longer sand—it becomes a pearl. As we begin to see diseases as irritants that need to be dealt with, we can go on about our lives (like the oyster) and incorporate the disease into our being in such a way that it is transformed and becomes a thing of beauty. In a similar way, our thoughts are like the soil upon which we build our foundation. We need to know that **what we think about and say to each other has an *actual* effect on us and others—physically, mentally, emotionally and spiritually.**

I had a friend years ago who would constantly greet a person with the statement: "You don't look a bit good." I have seen her teenage daughter come down the stairs feeling and looking healthy and full of life, then have her mother say to her: "You don't look a bit good." Immediately, her daughter began to look depressed, as if the energy were sucked right out of her. **This focus on what is *wrong* with us leads us away from what is *right* with us,** on both a personal and professional level. **Thoughts are things** and, when we say them aloud, we give them even more energy and strength. This young teenager would have been a healthier and better-adjusted person if her mother had greeted her in a positive way each morning. Starting the day in that way would have helped them *both* enjoy their lives in a more meaningful way.

When examining patients, if I saw from a patient's chart that she had ovarian cancer and then started treating the cancer, I might have missed who the patient was. It is quite possible that I would be so focused on the diagnosis (ovarian cancer) that I would hardly even notice the patient herself. I have had patients who, after sending them to a specialist, would come back and say: "I went to see him, and he never really talked to me." When I followed up with that specialist, he responded: "I spent fifteen to twenty minutes with her." The problem was that *he spent his time with my patient's* disease, *NOT with my* patient! This principle was driven home to me by the following story told to me by Elisabeth Kübler-Ross, MD[21] (the internationally-known author of *On Death and Dying*).

After she had a stroke, Elisabeth went with her son to see a neurologist. The neurologist proceeded to address her son, instead of her. This interchange lasted for about ten minutes before Elisabeth interrupted and, in her no-nonsense way, reminded the neurologist that she was *not* just a patient, she was a *person* and he was to talk to *her*—and if he continued to talk to her son, she would send her son out of the room! We frequently treat patients with diseases in this same way: by misdirecting our focus. In Living Medicine, if we find ourselves doing this, we call our focus immediately back to the patient—to the *person*—because **it is the physician and patient *together* that can bring the highest and best to the healing process.**

It is the rock of disease that needs to be destroyed, broken up and moved into the very foundation of our house of Living Medicine. As we examine these old concepts that are no longer working and need to be changed as we create the foundation of our new Living Medicine home, we get in touch with a deeper relationship with **Mother Earth**. It is she who **accepts our plan and recognizes the space that our being occupies within our *living* space on the earth.**

Another large boulder that we must deal with is the current concept of how to handle pain. In conventional medicine, *pain has become Enemy Number One in conjunction with any disease*. Rather than viewing pain as an indicator of an energy block that needs to be changed, it is regarded as *something that must be eliminated*. The Chinese concept of pain is that it represents a block in our *chi* (or

---

[21] Kübler-Ross, MD, Elisabeth. On Death and Dying: What the Dying Have to Teach Doctors, Nurses, Clergy and Their Own Families, 1969 (Re-issue Edition, 2014).

Life Force energy), and Chinese medicine physicians use acupuncture to remove that block and allow the *chi* energy to flow again. **If we are alive, we are going to have pain**, which means that we are connected to our nervous system and our very consciousness. I remember learning this principle as a seven-year-old child in India while riding in my father's Ford Model T, hearing the words: *"Buckshish, buckshish"* (which means "alms"), then turning around and looking into the face of a leper. This man did not frighten me, because I knew him. My parents worked with lepers, and he was one of the people in the leper colony. I knew the problem with leprosy was not pain—it was the opposite: the leper feels *no* pain, since the bacteria causing leprosy (*Mycobacterium leprae*) destroys nerve fibers. Lepers can put their hands in a fire and not know they are on fire, because they feel no pain. Rats can chew off their toes at night, and they will not know it. If my finger is cut off, the part that is severed does not feel *my* pain. Rather, the part of my hand connected with my nervous system feels my pain and alerts my body to the need to do something about it. **If I just stop the pain**, as in the disease process of leprosy, **then the corrective action is not taken.** Our concept of what pain is and how to deal with it presents a major boulder that must be moved and incorporated in its new form into the *living* process of creating the foundation of our new Living Medicine home.

There are also other rocks that need shifting. One is the way *medicine*, particularly during *my* learning years, *is still predominately male-dominated*. Not only were women a small minority within the health care system at that time, they were also ridiculed and ignored as much as possible. I went to the only women's medical college in the country at the time. *While there were fifty of us in the freshman class, only twenty-five of us graduated.* One of the reasons was that the faculty felt that we, as women physicians, needed to be stronger, better and more equipped than the men to deal with the field of medicine. Any lack of ability or stamina by a female physician would disqualify us to face "the man's world of medicine." The women surgeons I knew were tougher and more mannish than the men themselves, because they were told that was the only way they could succeed in medicine.

I started my internship at the Deaconess Hospital in Cincinnati. In all likelihood, I was given this position because my uncle was on the Board of Trustees of Deaconess Hospital. A woman physician had never preceded me in this position, so there was no place for me to stay, not even a room. For the nights when I was on call—and especially on weekend call, which was from Friday morning through Sunday night—my bed consisted of an X-ray table, a blanket and a pillow. I had no support or encouragement from the residents, particularly the surgical resident. He felt that women did not belong in medicine at all, and his job was to get me out. During this time, I became pregnant with my first child. This resident not only believed that women did not belong in medicine, he especially knew that *pregnant* women had no place in medicine! He gave me every difficult job he could, such as the long orthopedic surgical procedures that would start at 7:30 in the morning and last for four to five hours. Being pregnant put me at his mercy, and I had no recourse other than to show up without any breakfast, since there was no food available at that early hour in the hospital. I would hang on, literally, thinking at times that I would not make it through, and that both my baby and I would die. However, there was no way I was going to let him pronounce *that* sentence on us, so I hung in there. (I find it interesting that the child I was carrying during this time became an orthopedic surgeon!)

Then things began to change. I truly believe that **there are Universal forces that help us through difficult times and even angelic beings that can manifest as friends and helpers.** Suddenly, my schedule began to change. Instead of being scheduled for surgery at 7:30 AM, I was scheduled at nine o'clock and could then get something to eat before surgery. The resident confronted me on this and asked why I had changed the schedule…but *I* had not changed the schedule. Then one night, about three o'clock in the morning, as I returned to my X-ray table bed after seeing a patient, I saw that the tiny little housekeeper (Lucille) had pulled a chair up to the blackboard where the surgery schedule was listed. She was replacing my name at 7:30 AM with another intern's name and putting my name down in the nine o'clock spot! She literally became my personal angel. There were even times when I would get a call in the middle of the night and jump off my X-ray table to run for the phone that was down the hall. My pregnancy would catch up with me halfway there, and I would lose whatever I had eaten for dinner. Lucille would be right there, saying: "You just go right on, Dr. Gladys, I'll clean it up." And, bless her heart, she *did* clean it up, so I could go on with my work.

As years went by, the issues facing *women physicians* did not improve very much. In 1955, when my husband and I moved to Phoenix from Ohio, I was on the staff of Good Samaritan Hospital. The parking lot just south of the hospital was guarded by a huge man who was responsible for keeping that lot reserved strictly for physicians. Every time I parked there, I was confronted by him, as were the other women physicians. No matter what we did to try to identify ourselves as physicians, he simply could not comprehend it. We would hang our stethoscopes around our necks. We would swing them noticeably in front of us, as we walked. Some of the women physicians even wore their white coats. It did not make any difference. Every time he saw a woman parking in this lot, we would have to go through the whole process of identifying ourselves, showing our licenses and proving that we really were women doctors. This experience continued until the day a woman physician who was small in stature though great in spirit took charge. Betty Kilpatrick, MD was the kind of person who had the courage to preside over the births of my last two children, both of whom were born at home during a time when doing this was considered risky. When Betty, who stood just a little over five feet tall, was confronted by this huge obstacle of a guard, she barely came up to his umbilicus. Enough was enough! She took her stethoscope and began pounding on his belly. "There are fifteen women doctors in this city," she said. "We have a right to park here. You have no right to keep us out and you *will* let us park here." The poor man had no idea what was going on, because he could hardly see her under the round of his belly. After that incident, we had no problem parking our cars in the doctors' parking lot!

As women physicians, we have all faced situations like this and survived, not only because of our own inner strength and focus, but also because of the forces that support, guide and help *all* of us in such circumstances. **It is time to bring the *feminine* face of medicine**— which is the nurturing, caring aspect of love—**back into the practice of medicine.**

In the process of clearing the ground for our Living Medicine home, we come across *other concepts that simply need to be released*—like dirt that is superfluous and unusable—when preparing the ground upon which our new foundation will be laid. One such concept taught to us in medical school was that we should *never befriend our patients*, since this would cloud our judgment and make us unobjective. *This, I believe, is totally incorrect.* Some of my closest friends are people who started out as my patients. Because I got to know and love them, I have been more effective in working with them. As a matter of fact, *I think of all my patients as my friends.*

Another concept we learned in medical school was *never to give a patient false hope.* I do not believe there is such a thing. I believe *hope is a spiritual quality that embodies healing in its very essence.* I think **we can give false information, false expectation and false presentation; however,** we *never* **offer false hope. Sometimes, hope is the only thing that we *can* offer a patient.** We can share the hope of comfort in relationships, the hope of relief of some kind or even the hope of moving through the dying process with support.

The book *Selling Sickness*[22] by Ray Moynihan (a journalist and one of the world's leading health writers) and Allan Cassels (a Canadian policy researcher) illustrates *a* global *concept that needs to be released.* In it, the authors state that U.S. pharmaceutical companies have marketed their products to *healthy* people by using fear in their advertising techniques. This book goes into a great deal of detail

---

[22] Moynihan, Ray and Allan Cassels. *Selling Sickness - How Drug Companies Are Turning Us into Patients*, 2005.

to explain how the marketing strategies of the huge drug companies ("Big Pharma") have systematically and progressively transformed Life's *normal* maladies into major disease processes, turning worried-well[23,24] (or "healthy-unwell")[25,26] people into wounded-sick people. (Amazingly, Dr. Ann just informed me, the ICD-10 *now* has a diagnosis code for people with these labels:

Z71.1!) "Thus, shyness becomes a sign of 'social anxiety disorder' and pre-menstrual tension is turned into a mental illness, 'pre-menstrual dysphoric disorder.' Just being at risk of an illness has become a disease in its own right." *These normal, human conditions must be labeled as illnesses to be able to be charged for and billed to insurance companies for reimbursement.* These pharmaceutical companies advertise and attempt to sell drugs to the *consumer* using marketing campaigns to highlight medical conditions that may or may not be real, then recommend prescription medications as THE solution to treat the described conditions. Consumers then think they *need* the promoted drug. *When people make a direct link between a medical condition and a pharmaceutical, what may be a natural process then becomes a medical problem.* This exposé of Big Pharma further elaborates: "They [drug companies] claim that 90 percent of elderly people in the U.S. have a condition called 'high blood pressure,' that almost 50 percent of women in the U.S. have a sexual dysfunction called FSD, and that some 40 million U.S. citizens should be taking drugs to lower their cholesterol. With help from headline-hungry media, the latest condition is routinely described as widespread, severe, [critical] and always treatable with drugs." This kind of rhetoric is a promotional strategy for selling sickness and fear. Fear itself is a major cause of hypertension! **When fear enters our house of Liv-**

---

[23] Garfield, Sidney, MD (founder of Kaiser Permanente) coined this term in 1970 in an article that he wrote for Scientific American.

[24] Pontious, Michael J., MD. "Understanding the 'Worried Well'," J Fam Pract. 2002 January;51(1):30.

[25] Ramchandani, Dilip, MD et.al. "Meprobamate – Tranquilizer or Anxiolytic? A Historical Perspective," Psychiatric Quarterly, Vol 77, No 1, Spring 2006

[26] www.coursehero.com>file>psychiatrists-in-backwaters-of-psychiatry (p.9-11).

ing Medicine, it has the capacity and the ability to take over the entire building, because **when fear steps in, reason steps out.**

There is one rock that I see no way of *currently* eliminating. Everybody I know is dealing with it, and even though we have no solution for it right now, we are continuing to look for one. That rock is the issue of *insurance*—medical insurance, malpractice insurance and insurance of all types which have *all* come between the doctor and the patient, totally taking the focus of the healing process off of the patient and concentrating it on the disease and the modalities used to destroy the disease. There are many people trying to resolve this problem. **Insurance companies must stop separating the physician and the patient.** Somehow, *we must invent a new currency that is based on value for value, instead of one that is totally dependent on dollar for dollar.* Somehow, somewhere, this needs to be developed and become a reality, so that healing can really be a healing of the *total* person—body, mind and spirit. In the future, insurance is something that we will need to incorporate into our Living Medicine home. As time goes on, I believe that innovative solutions to the insurance crisis will reveal themselves, as we become more creative in our thinking and as people take more personal responsibility for their healing process. *The Physician Within each of us can and should play a part in discovering these innovative solutions.*

Since the field of Living Medicine represents a *living* process, **there will always be issues for which we have no apparent answers at the present time,** so **we need to keep our minds and hearts open for solutions.** Two examples follow of people that Dr. Ann and/or I personally know who did just that, and the world has been a better place because of the problems they solved and the solutions they came up with.

The first of these innovators was Cathy Kinnaird, RN (1951-2018). She was the person from whom Dr. Ann learned how to make flower essence remedies (FER) for her patients, especially emergency trauma solutions (ETS). The unique problem that Cathy solved was to create the *first* (and possibly *only*) flower essence pharmacy in existence at the time, where she offered *every flower essence producer in the world* the opportunity to have their product line in her pharmacy. That allowed "one-stop shopping" for anyone seeking these products, and she was always available to consult with whenever Dr. Ann had a difficult case where some rare or particular flower essence was needed to make the *exact* FER or ETS for a patient. A wealthy man purchased her flower essence pharmacy, then let it die...a truly sad outcome for us all. Perhaps someone who shares Cathy's passion, skill and vision will read these words and pick up where Cathy left off.

The second innovator is Col. Tim Kirk, USAF (Retired). As someone who experienced the trauma of war in the Middle East firsthand and returned from it with PTSD, he took on the challenge of discovering what it would take to decrease the national statistic of twenty-two veteran suicides per day. *His goal was to create a model that could be duplicated in every community in the country.* He has done that now in Sierra Vista, Arizona. In a sixteen-thousand square-foot building, he has brought together as many of the community's resources under one roof as possible which are willing to be a part of his vision. All a veteran has to do is "show up," and help is provided for whatever they need. He is currently in the process of writing the Warrior Healing Center[27] Operations Manual, so that this model can be duplicated in *any* community willing to take on this same challenge.

Both of these innovators are examples of what Dr. Ann calls the *real* "Johnny Appleseed" principle: *you can count the number of seeds in an apple, but not the number of apples in a seed.* **Never underestimate the power of *one* person to change the world.** This is why *individualized* medicine IS the foundation of Living Medicine, a concept which will be discussed at length in the next chapter.

When I built my own little house, we conducted a special house blessing after the dirt had been moved around in preparation for the foundation to be laid. Gathering friends and relatives, we created a time capsule into which we placed some precious things. My grandson put in plastic dinosaurs and Ninja Turtles, and each of us placed

---

[27] https://warriorhealingcenter.com

something that was important to us into the time capsule. After we buried it right where my library would be, we covered it and then sang and danced on the ground over it. In this way, we **created holy ground**. My prayer is that each one of us, as we create *our own* home of Living Medicine, will be able to personally consecrate it in such a way that it becomes *holy* ground. And, with our Living Medicine home built on *solid* ground, we will be claiming the promise in the Bible found in Matthew 7:24-25: "Everyone who hears these words of mine and acts on them will be like a man who built his house on rock. The rain fell, the floods came, and the winds blew and beat on that house, but *it did not fall*, because it had been founded on rock."

2

The Foundation

The next step in building our house of Living Medicine is to create a *solid and stable* foundation. It needs to be erected according to the master plan for that specific building, which includes the plumbing, electrical work and support structures. Plans for the rest of the edifice also need to be clear.

An ideal dwelling place does not require a perfect house. However, it must be constructed in harmony with our ideal or life purpose. If the materials used to create the foundation are not properly assembled, then the whole structure will find itself unable to withstand the life it was created to house. If there is too much sand and not enough cement or if there is a misuse of some of the ingredients that go into building the foundation, these defects will also cause instability in the structure. Likewise, if the foundation of our Living Medicine home is not built in harmony with our life purpose, it will not be strong enough to withstand the stresses and strains that inevitably come with the challenges and storms of life.

It is also essential that our foundation be in *precise* alignment with the master plan. It needs to be perfectly level, without a millimeter of discrepancy. The foundation must fit *exactly* into the earth and the environment on which it is being built. We must also take into consideration such things as weather (like heat and cold, rain and snow) in addition to whatever else Mother Nature offers in that specific environment.

As we build the foundation for our house of Living Medicine, we become aware of the reality that the foundation upon which *conventional* medicine has been built contains many shortcomings. To have our foundation be strong, we must identify some of these inadequacies and work with concepts that will help build a stronger and more sustainable foundation. Jesus said: "A house built on sand cannot stand" (Matthew 7:26-27). Much of what we have worked with in conventional medicine consists of sand. We now find ourselves in a situation in which *the* whole *system is broken.* Patients are unhappy with their care and often cannot get the attention and help they need and deserve. They are bewildered and confused, feeling abandoned much of the time. Physicians have become disillusioned. Many of them are unable to continue their practices because they cannot financially support themselves enough to even meet their basic needs. Some of them struggle with complete burnout and do not know where to turn.

In the world of impressive and exciting scientific programs, the *art* of medicine has been ignored, and many **physicians** have forgotten that they **are primarily *artists* who bring healing to the body.** Instead, most physicians have been taught to see themselves as *scientists*, abandoning the *art* of medicine in the caring for and understanding of the individual human being who needs help. *Science*, however, **should be a wonderful tool that can be utilized by the physician in his or her work and greatly enhance the** *art* **of medicine**, which taps into the healing energy of the patient.

Centuries ago, when musicians only had pipes and one-string instruments, they still produced beautiful music. However, when they perfected the violin and built a Stradivarius, musicians immeasurably upgraded their capability for moving the hearts of their listeners. In like manner, *science has taken the human need for healing,* which is comparable to the human need for music, *and moved it from its primitive condition to the promising present.* We now have instruments in conventional medicine *not* found in ages past that can be tuned and used. These instruments are constantly being improved and perfected. It takes training to learn to play the violin and a desire to spend untold number of hours practicing and perfecting this art. **The *art* of medicine requires** this same kind of **dedication and time to perfect** **it.** Both the science *and* the art of medicine require *constant and continuous practice* and an ongoing *commitment and effort* to grow and improve. Just as the violin is nothing without the violinist, **the *science* of medicine is nothing without the *art* of medicine. The physician must incorporate *both* into the healing process to function effectively.**

When my husband and I began studying acupuncture in the early 1970's, we were privileged to have two Japanese physicians as guests in our home. One evening they got into a heated discussion at the dinner table regarding acupuncture. The traditional physician insisted it was an *art* that, when properly practiced, could be therapeutic. His colleague, insisting that there had to be a scientific explanation for it, said it was necessary to evolve the *science* of acupuncture. It was a very exciting meal, especially since the discussion was all in Japanese, which neither of us understood! Our interpreter was a Catholic priest who had spent twenty years in Japan. It was then that we realized **both the science *and* the art of acupuncture are necessary.** East was East and West was West; in this instance, however, the two were about to meet. Our challenge, then, is to work toward accepting **science** as **a tool** that we can use **to practice our *art*** to the benefit of our fellow humans.

What is it that allows us to become artists? I believe the real answer to this question is *love*—the love of our Creator, who opens our hearts and minds to create scientific systems. These systems, in turn, like the beautiful violin, can be loved and used to bring into our lives and into the lives of our loved ones an attunement and an "at-one-ment." Paul reminds us in I Corinthians 13:13 (italics are mine): "Now abideth faith, hope and love, and *the greatest of these is love*." It is our training and tools that allow us as physicians to show this love, in our own *unique* ways, to our fellow human beings, including our patients.

Neither music nor medicine amounts to anything, however, without the appropriate *audience* to benefit from the performance of the art. **The physician needs the patient, and the patient needs the physician—one is *not* complete without the other.** Because **COMMUNICATION is the *central principle* of the *art* of medicine,** *becoming an* effective *communicator is* essential *for* all *physicians who want to become skilled in the ART of medicine.* So it seems obvious that *teaching* effective communication skills ought to be a part of *every* medical school curriculum. Some medical schools recognize the value of this principle and have been including it in their curriculum for years.[28,29] Others are just beginning to move in the right direction regarding this important principle.

Medicine has evolved more and more as a *science* and less and less as an *art*. We have developed amazing scientific tools with which to fight disease. Even the concept of medicine as an *art* has been ridiculed. If something did not have a scientific basis, it was not considered worth looking at or researching further. We, as physicians, were taught that disease and pain were our enemies, and our job in life was to attack and get rid of them. Science became our god, and the spiritual nature of the human being was sacrificed to that god. For me, this is a struggle that never quite resolved itself until the concept of Living Medicine was given to me. The medicine I believed in and knew that I needed to be part of since I was a toddler was an *art* in which science would serve as a magnificent tool. What I learned in medical school, however, was that medicine is a *science* that gave me tools with which to fight disease and kill pain.

When I got deeply involved in the practice of medicine as it intertwined with the lives of my patients, I began to look at this concept in a more objective way, so that I could compare the science and the art of medicine. What I found was that, in science, we are expected to do double-blind, placebo-controlled studies. Without such studies, our research is considered invalid and useless. Yet, *in the art of medicine, we find that **no two individuals are alike**, and **no two disease***

---

[28] Neufeld, VR and Barrows, HS. "The 'McMaster Philosophy': an approach to medical education," J Med Educ, 1974;49(11):1040-1050.

[29] https://mdprogram.mcmaster.ca>mcmaster-md-program

processes are exactly alike, **either**—just as no two cancers are *exactly* alike, even if their diagnoses are called by the same name. Nor do individuals react to medications or other treatment modalities in *exactly* the same way. **Any one** of us **may respond to** *any* **kind of treatment differently at different times and stages** in our lives. *The tool of double-blind, placebo-controlled studies in research is useful; however, it is* not *infallible.* Such studies give us information, yet, as in any art, we then need to be able to apply this information *uniquely,* moment to moment, with every individual, *in conjunction with* the *ART* of healing.

In the *science* **of medicine, everything must be tested. In the** *art* **of medicine, it must be practiced.** As in any art, for instance, playing the piano, music must be learned and understood. The instrument must be worked with, as well as tuned, for its quality of sound and ability to produce the music. The pianist must also practice, taking the tools that have been learned, and work with them until the pianist perfects his or her art. The same pianist can play "Chopsticks" or a Beethoven symphony. Physicians also know that they must practice and thus we call what we do the *practice* of medicine, as we learn and understand *our* scientific tools and how they can benefit each patient.

In the *science* of medicine, the physician does not get involved emotionally with the patient. Medical school teaches us to be observant and not allow our feelings to interfere with our practice. **In the** *art* **of medicine,** however, **there must be a deep engagement of the physician-as-therapist with the patient.** It is only then that the observations we have made and the information we have gathered with our scientific tools can be used to deal with and help that *specific* person. *The therapist part of us thus becomes an equally important part of the healing team, as we are transformed from being just an observer watching from the sidelines into the healer we can become.*

In the *science* of medicine, the physician is trained to be a doctor. We learn how to diagnose and treat diseases. **In the** *art* **of medicine, physicians need to become educated in the** *use* **and** *application* **of the training they have received.** *You can train a pet, however,* *you need to educate a child.* To do either task effectively, though, requires engaging the sentience of each *individual* being, human or animal.

In the *science* of medicine, it is almost as if we are artists being taught to paint-by-number. This color goes with this number, this color goes in that spot. The design has been laid out. The therapy must be done in a certain way. **In the *art* of medicine, there must be variety. There is no pattern that is laid down.** Artists find the *creative spark* within themselves and can put that on any kind of tangible media. The physician needs that same creative spark when practicing the *art* of medicine. It cannot be a "treat-by-number" process. **The tools can be *exactly* the same in the art and science of medicine. Engaging the spark of creativity within *both* the patient and the physician when utilizing those tools,** however, **is what brings Life to the healing process.**

I once spoke with a neuroscientist from Pfizer, Inc. in Connecticut. He called me because he was doing some deep soul-searching regarding some of the definitive research he was conducting on Alzheimer's disease. Having been interested in the Edgar Cayce material for years, he felt that some of Cayce's concepts about the sympathetic and parasympathetic nervous systems, in conjunction with osteopathic craniosacral manipulation, might be right on target. However, these concepts clashed with the approach taken by his company. I talked to him about his intentions and suggested to him that his *focus* was what was most important, and that holistic medicine *could* include what he was doing with his pharmaceutical research. Furthermore, I also reminded him that his being in the center of the scientific community could bring light into that community. We talked about the concept of Living Medicine and that, if he focused on Living and Life rather than on destroying Alzheimer's disease, he could continue doing the work he considered so important *and* feel better about his contribution to healing patients with this disease. This story serves as a beautiful example of how **the art and science of medicine work *together* to create Living Medicine, so that Life itself**

becomes the medicine. *My prayer is that the huge temples of the science of medicine, which we call hospitals and research centers, will find themselves bowing to the temple of the* art *of medicine, which is the human body*. In the milieu of the current pandemic that is present in the world as we write this second edition, where the *science* of medicine is being looked to for providing *all* the answers to solving this problem, the *art* of medicine is being both ignored and corrupted. At a time when humans need to rely on each other the most, they are ignoring what is good for the *we* in the process of taking care of the *me*, choosing fear and power over Love and Life. Yet, it is **Love and Life** that **leads to health and healing**, both individually and globally. "We are all in this together" is the phrase that we keep hearing, which means that *we have to learn to take care of ourselves* in the process of *taking care of others, instead of at their* expense. We must remember that we are individual cells in the body of the world, and we need *all* of the cells to thrive for the body to be able to heal fully and completely.

To have a solid foundation for our Living Medicine home, *we must find the* proper *balance between art and science, in addition to the proper relationship between the body, mind and spirit*. The Cayce readings say: "The spirit is the life; the mind is the builder; the physical is the result."[30] The metaphor that I use to relate to this affirmation is that of an old slide projector, which is the Spirit or the Light or Life. The mind represents the slide placed in that projector, and the physical is the screen upon which the picture on the slide is projected. In conventional medicine, we have spent a great deal of time and most of our energy on what is projected onto the screen or the body. There is nothing wrong with that. If the screen (body) is broken, dirty or unclear, then what is projected onto it cannot really be understood and needs to be clarified. In other-than-conventional medicine, we have also spent a lot of time working with the mind and the effect it has on the physical body. We are now aware that **the mind is a pivotal component in the functioning of the body**. Since biofeedback demon-

---

[30] www.edgarcayce.org. Reading 900-70.

strated the interrelationship of the mind and the body, this relationship has become part of the *science* of medicine, and it is now readily accepted that **both are integral to the whole healing process**. *The field of holistic medicine was born when physicians began to realize that, **without the** spiritual **component in medicine, we were missing the heart of the healing process**.* As with the slide projector, it does not matter how clear the slide is or how usable the screen is; if the projector is unplugged from its Source, which is the activating energy of Life itself, nothing will project onto the screen!

I think I became aware of this principle as a nine-year-old child in India when I woke up one morning, sat straight up in bed and said to myself: "Gladys, there's something wrong in this world. You don't have a friend." This was true. I am a Sagittarius and, if people made me angry, I punched them out and dealt with my anger in an aggressive way. I had brothers from whom I learned to fight, which extended into my relationships with other people. I thought: "I don't like the way I feel. And, if I'm fighting all the time, that doesn't make me feel good. Who do I know that doesn't look at Life this same way?" The obvious person was my mother. She was the kind of person who could take anything that came her way and, with just a minor shift in presenting and reframing the situation, could come up with a humorous outlook. When she was eighty-nine years old, she fell and broke her left knee and the ribs on her left side. My father and I were moving her from the gurney onto the X-ray table when she looked up, saw the pain on our faces and said: "The old gray mare ain't what she used to be." The next day she died. In 2020, I found myself in a similar situation, in this *same* hospital, and I did *not* die, even though I was reminded that most people of my age *usually* do not survive such injuries. You can imagine how surprised everyone was when I spent only one night in the ICU and was discharged only two days later!

I had lived with my mother's kind of gentle humor and recognized the difference that it made, because my mother had friends all over the world. People loved her and respected her. I thought I would much rather be like *her* than the way I was, so I started to change. I told myself that I was going to laugh instead of fight. Basically, I took that slide from the projector that said I was a mean, nasty, hateful kid and I either cleaned it up or threw it away. Then, I replaced it with one that said: "You're going to laugh. You're not going to fight everything or everyone that comes your way." *Doing that one thing completely changed my life.* By the time I was a senior in high school, I was labeled the class clown!

As a recent centenarian, I now realize that my sudden awareness of having no friends ninety years ago may have been my first **"aha" moment**. From our discussion about this moment in my life, Dr. Ann shared with me her definition of an "aha" moment that she learned from someone whose insight and wisdom she greatly admires like I admire Edgar Cayce: Stephen Covey.

Although no one knows *exactly* how "aha" moments come about, what we *do* know is that the components of having one almost universally look like this (italics are mine): **"Suddenly, I *saw* things differently, and because I saw differently, I *thought* differently, I *felt* differently, I *behaved* differently."**[31] As a result of this understanding, Dr. Ann committed herself to creating a medical practice based on *being* with patients in such a way that their having "aha" moments about their health issues became one of her major goals. Consequently, the compliance rate of the patients in her practice with their *co-created treatment plans* became consistently ninety percent or better...just like I was able to finally feel successful in creating friends in my life as a result of my "aha" moment as a nine-year-old. *It is definitely a principle in Living Medicine that has stood the test of time*, even though neither of us had that awareness at the time. I suppose that's why it is said that "hindsight is *always* 20/20!"[32] (italics are mine)

To function at all, the projector needs to be connected to its source (electricity). It was my connection with my source, which was my mother's love and sense of humor, that led me to go beyond my

[31] Covey, Stephen. The 7 Habits of Highly Effective People, 1989.

[32] Menand, Louis. In "Notable Quotables," a book review of The Yale Book of Quotations, www.newyorker.com (Feb 11, 2007), this quote was attributed to Billy Wilder.

anger and reactivity and connect on a deep level to my *Divine Source.* Once *that* connection became real in my life, I was able to look at people and situations from a completely different perspective. *It is this principle of recognizing the spiritual aspect of a person's life to be* at least *as important as the physical and mental aspects that may* most *differentiate holistic medicine from conventional medicine.*

For years I lectured on the importance of distinguishing *the differences between the science and the art of medicine.* The following chart is an example of some of these differences:

SCIENCE ....ART
Energy of the mind ....Energy of the heart
Double-blind studies....................Each individual is unique
Facts...Imagination and creativity
Statistics and numbers................Individuals are not numbers
Results (static............................Ongoing learning (dynamic)
Measured in finite time ....Subject to infinite change
Can be taught............................Must be experienced

Both the science and the art of medicine are important. We need to understand *first* what we have been taught (science) to learn what we *truly* need to learn to help ourselves and our patients *heal* (art), instead of settling for just becoming symptom-free.

The process of bringing back into the *heart* of medicine what it takes to *truly* heal has presented the field of medicine with a major challenge. The predominant aspects of what it takes to do that (the energy of the feminine, the *art* of medicine, the spirit of alternative modalities, the physician/patient partnership and the awareness that we are *total* beings—body, mind and spirit) has resulted in the need to come up with terms that are more descriptive than "other-than-conventional." For example, when physicians realized that using conventional medicine *alone* limited their access to available healing modalities from around the world, the term **complementary** *medicine*[33] came into being. When physicians began using other-than-conventional modalities (e.g. homeopathy, herbal medicine, acupuncture and biofeedback) *instead of* conventional medical treatments, we labeled it *alternative medicine*. *Traditional medicine* became a term when physicians realized that conventional medicine was a relatively *new* addition to their therapeutic armamentarium, and that certain aspects of medicine (such as massage, prayer, color and song) have been used since the beginning of time. It is specifically defined as "the sum total of knowledge, skills and practices based on the theories, beliefs and experiences *indigenous to different cultures* that are used to maintain health as well as to prevent, diagnose, improve or treat physical and mental illnesses."[34] My earliest contribution to these shifting paradigms involved redefining the *physician/patient partnership* as "contacting the Physician Within," a concept about which Jess Stearn and I wrote an entire book.[35] When it became apparent that the practice of medicine failed to address the *spiritual* nature of our humanness—and recognize the triune nature of our being as body, mind and spirit—a small group of five physicians came up with the term *"holistic medicine,"* and the American Holistic Medical Association (AHMA)[36] was born. This new paradigm acknowledged that, **for *true* healing to take place, there must be a recognition of the *spiritual* nature of our beings.** The *feminine face of medicine*, however, was still practically nonexistent back then (mid-1970's). For example, I was the only female physician among that group of five physicians who co-founded the AHMA, just as Dr. Ann was the only female physician among the group of five physicians from the AHMA who co-founded the American Board of Holistic Medicine almost twenty years later (1995-2000). It wasn't until 2003 that the National Library of Medicine put together the traveling exhibition (retired in 2012) *Changing the Face of Medicine: Celebrating*

---

[33] www.medicinenet.com>complementary>and>alternative>medicine.

[34] www.sciencedirect.com>topics>traditional>medicine>an>overview.

[35] McGarey, Gladys T., MD with Jess Stearn. The Physician Within You, 2000.

[36] www.ncbi.nlm.nih.gov>pmid14619031.

America's Women Physicians[37] that women began to get recognized in the medical profession for their contributions.

Holistic medicine was and still is dedicated to reawakening the *art* of medicine, as well as recognizing its importance in the healing process. Although it has done better than most other-than-conventional forms of medicine with acknowledging the contributions of women physicians, it still struggles at times with giving more than lip service to holding women physicians as *fully* equal to their male counterparts. However, this paradigm remains *strongly* committed to bringing about the sorely needed integration of the triune nature of our being (body, mind and spirit) within both ourselves *and* our patients. *Living Medicine goes beyond this.* Living Medicine brings together the concepts that **Life itself is the healer,** and that **Life itself is what *truly* brings the body, mind and spirit into balance.** Thus, *Life itself is* the *basic ingredient on which the foundation of Living Medicine is built.*

There are many ways to work with our spiritual nature. For example, even a surgical procedure conducted in a manner of caring and understanding *can* be an awakening experience. The following story demonstrates how Living Medicine can be used in a surgical setting.

I once had a patient in the office who told me that, when she had a very serious surgery many years earlier, the young resident came in to discuss with her what was to be done. He explained how *she* could contribute to her healing process and then took a little quiet time with her before the surgery. The whole experience was a time of spiritual growth and beauty for this woman and became a turning point in her life. **It is not that we have neglected to use our tools as physicians with expertise, it is the spirit with which these tools are *used* that makes all the difference.**

The concept of Living Medicine does not eliminate the basic scientific information that we were taught in medical school. It is important to have a solid foundation—solid in anatomy and physiology, microbiology, neurology, gastroenterology and so forth. It is also important

---

[37] https://www.nlm.nih.gov>exhibtions.

to understand the body's involvement in the process of disease: the microbial component; the way in which the immune system interacts with invasive pathological organisms; how medications affect the disease process; what the disease itself is, as well as how the body responds to it; and to know about and understand the medications that affect the disease processes. If our foundation is going to be solid, we also need to make sure that we understand the ways in which disease processes affect our very lives. ***Conventional* medicine brings its knowledge to Living Medicine, and Living Medicine infuses this knowledge with Life.**

The science and art of medicine come together very clearly when dealing with issues of the endocrine system. The medical science of endocrinology has made giant steps in understanding how the endocrine system functions in our body. We are just beginning to appreciate how it is connected to and associated with our emotional responses. We understand the connections that our thoughts and choices have on the actual functioning of the endocrine system, just as the products of this system have an impact on our thoughts and choices. This two-way exchange can occur because *the endocrine glands are neuro-hormonal transducers.* In other words, they receive input from the sensory nervous system and then translate that information into hormonal activity. For example, we now know that with the use of biofeedback, a person can have some control over the activity of the adrenals, which in turn helps maintain blood pressure and heart rate. This is also more or less true of the other endocrine glands, depending on how much control the individual has over his or her own thoughts, choices and emotions. The Hindu fakir (holy man), for example, can slow his physiological functions down to such a minimal level that he can be pronounced dead and maintain that status for many hours. This has been validated by two researchers, Alyce and Elmer Green, PhD in their groundbreaking work with biofeedback.[38]

---

[38] Green, Elmer, PhD and Alyce. Beyond Biofeedback – The Science of Consciousness, 1977. Out of print. A pdf copy of the book can be downloaded from www.consciousnessandbiofeedback.org.

The *scientific* aspect of the endocrine system continues to be researched to understand the delicate balance of this system. Medications (e.g. bio-identical hormone replacement therapy, including thyroid hormone) and external devices (e.g. the Brain State headband and other biofeedback systems) have been developed to help us clarify the *physiological* nature of this system. For example, from the classic *Williams Textbook of Endocrinology*[39] to the work of Broda Barnes, MD[40] (1906-1988), Mark Starr, MD,[41] Denis Wilson, MD[42] and even the medical medium Anthony William,[43] all speak to the impact of thyroid hormone on *every* cell of the body. In particular, Broda Barnes, MD's *epidemiological studies* involving an extensive analysis of seventy-thousand autopsy records of people who died in Graz, Austria between 1930 and 1970, showed thyroid deficiency to be THE *common denominator* in susceptibility to infection, coronary artery disease, arthritis, diabetes, lung cancer and emphysema in up to forty percent of that population.[44] Interestingly, in that research, the measurement of *basal body temperature*[45] was found to be *significantly more reliable* than laboratory testing to determine the presence or absence of the need for thyroid replacement therapy. In addition, other research in iodine deficiency[46] and the best way to test for it[47] has since been done that further supports Dr. Barnes' findings.

---

[39] 14th edition, published 2019.

[40] Barnes, Broda O., MD and Galton, Lawrence. Hypothyroidism: The Unsuspected Illness, 1976 and www.brodabarnes.org (research foundation).

[41] Starr, Mark, MD. Hypothyroidism Type 2: The Epidemic, 2013 (6th edition, revised).

[42] Wilson, E. Denis, MD. Wilson's Thyroid Syndrome: A Reversible Thyroid Problem, 2001 (4th edition) and the Doctor's Manual for Wilson's Temperature Syndrome, 2005.

[43] William, Anthony. Medical Medium: Thyroid Healing, 2017.

[44] www.medical-library.net>broda-barnes. Article by Ron Kennedy, MD.

[45] https://headsuphealth.com>blog>basal>body>temperature>tracking>part>one>thyroid and www.integratedhealth.com>barnes>axial>temperature>test

[46] Brownstein, David, MD. Iodine: Why You Need It, Why You Can't Live Without It, 2014 (5th ed.) and Overcoming Thyroid Disorders, 2008 (3rd ed.) and Salt Your Way to Health, 2009.

[47] Fletchas, Jorge D. MD. "Orthoiodosupplementation in a Primary Care Practice," www.optimox.com>iodine-study-10 and https://www.youtube.com/watch?v=VvEj1YYWvR0 and www.hakalalabs.com.

To practice the *art* of medicine using science as a tool, it is important that we also look at the endocrine system from the point of view of our *spiritual* nature. As we become aware of the symbolism associated with the endocrine system as it relates to our spiritual nature, we can then contact our unconscious self through dreams and visions.

Our Life Force has been known in religious terms as spirit, *chi*, prana and kundalini. Each of these terms represents *the rising energy that activates the spiritual centers*, also known as *chakras* in the Hindu tradition, the *seven stars/lampstands/spirits/candlesticks/ churches* in the New Testament (Revelations, chapters 1-3) and *Ezekiel's Wheel* in the Old Testament (Ezekiel 10:9-10). These vortices of energy in specific areas of the body are *the energetic outpicturings of the seven major endocrine glands*. These glands represent **the seven spiritual centers**. The *first chakra* is represented by the testicles and ovaries where the sperm and ovum are created. The *second chakra* is represented by the Leydig cells (the interstitial cells in the testicles and ovaries which produce the sex hormones). The adrenal glands represent the *third chakra*, which is known as the major energy center. They sit like little caps on top of the kidneys. The *fourth chakra* is in the thymus gland, which is the heart chakra (also known as the love center), located in the chest cavity. The *fifth chakra* is in the neck and is represented by the thyroid gland, which is associated with the will. The *sixth chakra* is represented by the pineal gland and lies in the center of the brain. It is associated with light and regulates all the body's cycles. The *seventh chakra* is represented by the pituitary gland and lies a little below and in front of the pineal gland. It is the master gland and controls all the other endocrine glands. Each one of these glands has been uniquely identified and symbolized in different cultures throughout time.

*The four chakras that are located within the trunk of the body are known as **the earth centers**.* The symbolism associated with these chakras has to do with *four elements* in the following order: *earth* with the first chakra, *water* with the second, *fire* with the third and *air* with the fourth. *They also are represented by animals*: the *bull or* the *cow* represents the first chakra, the *androgynous man* represents the second, the *lion or* the *cat* represents the third and the *eagle* represents the fourth. Different cultures have different symbols associated with these four chakras.

The five senses tie the earth centers to the centers in the heavens. The relationships of these five senses to the chakra system are: the first chakra is the sense of *smell*; the second chakra is the sense of *taste*; the third chakra is *sight*; the fourth chakra is the sense of *feeling*; and the fifth chakra is the sense of *hearing*. The two higher chakras come into this symbolism as we look at the seven notes of the piano, the seven colors of the rainbow, the seven days of the week and so forth. In her book *Anatomy of the Spirit,*[48] Carolyn Myss (PhD researcher and internationally-acclaimed medical intuitive) goes into great detail about how this system works. Two other books offer greater detail about the functioning and the symbolism associated with the chakra system.[49,50] Many more books have also been written that deal with this subject.

It is important to be aware of the *symbolism associated with the endocrine glands* because we use this symbolism in our everyday lives. Our dreams, if we are going to interpret them at all, have a deeper and more useful language when we incorporate our understanding of the symbols associated with the chakras. For instance, dreaming about a *lion or* a *tiger* provides a symbol of *adrenal* activity. If we dream of an *eagle or* a *hummingbird*, we are connecting with the activity of the *thymus*. It is very helpful in working with people's dreams to understand some of these metaphors as illustrated by the following case history.

A patient of mine had a series of dreams about a tiger. He was having a hard time controlling his temper, and his blood pressure

---

[48] Carolyn Myss, PhD. Anatomy of the Spirit: The Seven Stages of Power and Healing, 1996.

[49] McGarey, Gladys T. MD. Budhu's Path to Enlightenment, 2006.

[50] Kunz, Dora. The Personal Aura, 1991.

was high. When he began relating his dreams to me, he first saw a tiger that was locked up in his basement that had to be fed. He had several dreams dealing with this tiger. Then he dreamed he was holding onto the tiger's tail. He had allowed the tiger to come out of the basement, and it was pulling him down a cinder path. His feet were bleeding, but he held on tightly to the tiger's tail. Soon thereafter, he dreamed he was in Oak Creek Canyon in Sedona, Arizona, splashing in the water with the tiger. This dream series took place over a period of years, during which he was working with his emotions, meditating, doing yoga and biofeedback, in addition to paying attention to his diet. He was learning not only to control his anger but also his blood pressure, which he did *without* having to use blood pressure medication!

There has probably never been a point in time that we have known as much about the body and the mind, as well as their diseases, than we do at the current time. We now understand a great deal about how emotions interact with and impact the body, mind and spirit of an individual. We have research at our fingertips that represents solid science and good medicine. There is no country in the world where acute illnesses, trauma, surgical procedures and chemical intervention are as well-studied and practiced as in the United States. If I have a major trauma, such as a broken leg, there is no place I would rather be for my therapy than in our United States. *The question is: how can we make these ART of medicine tools available to all people and not just physicians?*

During a magazine interview in August 2002, the writer asked me: "How should the state of Arizona contend with the shortage of skilled medical professionals?" My answer was: "The way to deal with the lack of medical care in this state is by empowering individuals to take back their power to participate in their own healing process, by allowing *each one* to contact and work with *their own* Physician Within in *whatever* way that works uniquely for them. They know what they can and cannot eat. They know exercise is healthy and worthwhile. The only way we can do this is *by empowering the individual*, because we're never going to have enough doctors to conquer all the diseases." *This holds true to this day.*

If the field of medicine is really going to move *effectively* into the future, we each need to take responsibility for ourselves. We need to stop blaming other people for anything and everything that happens to us. We need to work with physicians as partners and truly allow *healing* to happen. *The importance of* each person *accepting responsibility for his or her own healing is a major ingredient in blending science with the* art *of medicine.* The following story illustrates this point, I think, very well.

Years ago, I had a patient call me on a Friday afternoon from Flagstaff, Arizona. At the time, I was living in Casa Grande, Arizona— a forty-five-minute drive from my office. Since it was late in the afternoon, I decided to wait until I got home to return her call. When I got home, I couldn't find the message, so I thought I would just wait until Monday to call her back. If she were really in trouble, I assumed she would probably call me over the weekend. On Monday, when I got back to the office and found her message, I called her. She said: "I was really angry with you when you didn't call me back, but then I got to thinking: 'If Dr. Gladys had called me back, she probably would have said: What do *you* think is wrong?' I probably would have said: 'I think I have a bladder infection, but the doctor said I have a vaginal infection.'" With this information in mind, she went back to her doctor on Saturday, telling him she thought she had a bladder infection. When he *again* said he thought she had a vaginal infection, she asked him to check *again* and, of course, *she* was right! So, you see, *when she checked with the Physician Within herself, she got information that the Physician Without did* not *have*, and they were then able to work together as a team to solve her *actual* problem. To me, it is imperative to teach our medical students and residents that **those of us who have the credentials to be called physicians can only find our *real* colleague (the Physician Within the *patient*) when we treat that colleague with respect, have an *open mind* and an *open heart*, with *no ego attachment to the outcome* of that col-**

league's/patient's problem *other than to be of service* **to his or her well-being.** Not understanding this principle may not impact the patient in a *major way—though it could*—as the following story[51] Dr. Ann shared with me illustrates so well (bold is ours):

> *Two battleships assigned to the Training squadron had been at sea on maneuvers in heavy weather for several days. I was serving on the lead battleship and was on watch on the bridge as night fell. The visibility was poor with patchy fog, so the captain remained on the bridge, keeping an eye on all activities. Shortly after dark, the lookout on the wing of the bridge reported: 'Light, bearing on the starboard bow.' 'Is it steady or moving astern?' the captain called out. Lookout replied: 'Steady, captain,' which meant we were on a dangerous collision course with that ship. The captain then called to the signalman: 'Signal that ship: We are on a collision course, advise you change course 20 degrees.' Back came a signal: 'Advisable for* ***you*** *to change course 20 degrees.' The captain said: 'Send: I'm a captain. Change course 20 degrees.' 'I'm a seaman second class,' came the reply. 'You had better change course 20 degrees.' By that time, the captain was furious. He spat out: 'Send: I'm a battleship. Change course 20 degrees.' Back came the flashing light: 'I'm a lighthouse.* ***We changed course.****'*

As physician "captains," **we must leave our egos at the door when we are with our** "seaman second class" (or any other rank) **patients,** especially when *their* Physician Within is firmly and respectfully press-

---

[51] Covey, Stephen. The 7 Habits of Highly Successful People, 1989.

ing to get our attention. Otherwise, we could end up having a "dangerous collision course" outcome with them instead of a healing journey. Another story that comes to mind to illustrate this principle involves my oldest son (Carl) who has been a retired orthopedic surgeon for many years now. When he had finished his training and was ready to start his practice, he said to me: "Mom, I'm really worried. Here I am with all this training, and I am going out to work with people. I'll have people's lives in my hands, and I don't know if I can handle the responsibility." Having struggled with this same problem for years, I was able to answer him: "Son, as a physician, *you* may pull an incision together and suture it well, but *you* cannot make it heal. If you think *you* are the one who does the healing, you *should* be scared. If you can understand, however, that **you are *just one* of the channels through whom healing moves**; that ***your* job is to contact the Physician Within *each* person to awaken the healing force in *them***; and, if you do the very best job you know how to do, then you have nothing to fear." (We teach our children what we need to learn!)

I could have also told my orthopedic surgeon son that **the most important question to ask *every* patient** to begin the process of healing is this one: **Why do you want to get well?** *The patient's answer to this question will always lead you to where you need to focus as their physician.* In addition, I could have likewise told him that **an important follow-up question** to this first one **is: "What do you want to get well for?** Is it to go right back to doing the things that made you sick in the first place, or are you ready to make a change in your life and *fully* commit yourself to the healing process, which means to begin the journey of becoming in harmony with your *total* being—mind, body and spirit?" Even though *these are* not *the questions that are currently taught to our physicians-in-training* to ask of their patients, I believe that they are **two of the most important questions** to teach them, if they are **to learn the *art* as well as the science of medicine.**

In Dr. Ann's practice, she started out asking her patients the following question which she learned from her classes with Stephen Covey: **"What one thing could you do in your personal and pro-**

fessional life that, if you did it on a regular basis, would make a tremendous positive difference in your life?"[52] From there, she developed a definition of **optimal health** as being **"soul-satisfying" work + "soul-satisfying" partnership**. Reading the results of the Cuber and Haroff study[53] and putting it together with some statistics on work satisfaction,[54] divorce and relationship dissolution[55] led her to this definition.

In summary, Dr. Ann found that the data revealed that eighty-five percent of people get up and go to work every day to a job that they really do *not* like *at all*; they do it because they have "to keep food on the table." Ten percent of people have the kind of work that, to them, is "just ok." They stay in their job for one of three reasons: because of the benefits they receive from doing so; they are marking time "until something better comes along"; or until retirement (and a pension) is imminent, etc. *Only five percent of people work at a job they really love*, one that "makes their heart sing." The statistics regarding relationships were even worse: ninety-five percent, five percent and one percent, respectively. *Those that were healthiest*, Dr. Ann concluded, were those *in the five percent category for work and the one percent category for partnership*, for which she coined the term "soul-satisfying."

This concept has long been a principle in her medical practice that she discusses with her patients from the outset. If she finds that her patients are struggling in either of these areas, she makes two immediate recommendations: career counseling that includes testing[56] and/or learning the *Imago Dialogue*,[57] a communication model that was co-created by the husband and wife team of Harville Hendrix, PhD and Helen LaKe-

---

[52] Covey, Stephen. The 7 Habits of Highly Successful People, 1989.

[53] Cuber, J.F. (with Haroff, P.B.). Sex and the Significant Americans: A Study of Sexual Behavior Among the Affluent , 1966.

[54] www.ReturnToNow.net>2017/09/22>85%>of>people>hate>their>jobs>gallup>poll >says.

[55] Fine, Mark A. and Harvey, John H, editors. Handbook of Divorce and Relationship Dissolution, 2013.

[56] 16-PF, Strong Vocational Interest Inventory, MMPI (or equivalent).

[57] www.imagorelationshipswork.com.

38

lly Hunt, PhD. Simply put, it is *an "intentional" dialogue that is taught to create connection and empathy.* While it has been used *predominantly* with couples, Dr. Ann's mentors[58] are now also using it to enhance effective communication in families of *all* kinds, as well as in the workplace.

Dr. Ann also learned from one of her medical school professors early on not to "skimp" on taking a medical history, "because **the patient** *always* **knows what's wrong with them**. If you give them [their Physician Within] a chance to tell you by *really* listening to them, you will find out more than any test or exam can ever tell you about what's *really* going on with them."[59]

This advice paralleled another principle she also learned from Stephen Covey years before she went to medical school: "**Listen twice as much as you speak**,"[60] as well as the fifth of the "five L's " (listening) of Living Medicine, discussed in detail in the upcoming library chapter. Dr. Ann still does this kind of medical history to this day, based on an open-ended set of questions that she gives the patient in the new patient packet on her website.[61] She said that the longest history she ever had a patient bring to their first visit was eighty pages, single-spaced! The shortest one was a blank sheet of paper.

The foundation of our Living Medicine home remains very fragile and undependable until we grapple with and address the issue of the physician/patient relationship and then *observe and experience* the physician truly *becoming* a coach in the healing process. When I was president of the American Holistic Medical Association in 1984, I wrote an article that I am quoting here in its entirety, as it is no longer in print. I believe it captures *the ingredients that strengthen this important aspect of creating a strong foundation*, so that our work in the future will be right in line with, working with and responding to the changes that are coming in this quickly-evolving world of health and healing.

---

[58] www.mayakolman.com.

[59] Henderson, Bryn J. DO/JD. www.regenerativemedgroup.com

[60] Covey, Stephen. The 7 Habits of Highly Successful People, 1989.

[61] www.nonprotocolmedicine.com.

*In September of this year [1984], I was in London for the formation of the British Holistic Medical Association meeting. While there, I met physicians from many different countries. One of the physicians was an orthopedic surgeon from South Africa. As we were talking about various things, he said something which stuck with me, which I would like to share with you. He said the motto in his office was what he called **the three A's**: **accessibility, affability and ability**. It was important for everybody from his front desk on back to know and understand these three A's.*

*The concept of **ACCESSIBILITY** is truly basic in a holistic practice. If we are not available to our patients, if our actual hours and our lifestyle is such that patients cannot get to us, then there isn't very much that we can do to help them. Beyond that, accessibility to me means being willing to allow a patient to access more than our time, even more than our knowledge. We must allow them to be[come] part of the essence of our unique healing quality: the spirit within. Without accomplishing this goal, we have not really made contact with the patient. We may have bound up their wounds and given them some relief from their symptoms; but until we are really available to them, we cannot work in the area of true healing. Recall that **Mother Teresa had to become accessible to the outcasts in Calcutta before her mission became a reality**. In order to do this, she felt that she had to go and live as they lived, becoming part of their* whole life *as much as she could. We may not need to do what Mother Teresa did. At some level of our awareness, however, we do need to be accessible to our patients at a deeper level than just a passing relationship, if we are to really be able to truly help them heal.*

AFFABILITY. Physicians might be accessible to their patients on a physical level yet be so caught up with their own problems or issues that they don't even understand the importance of kindness and gentleness and the qualities of spirit which separate us from animals and make us truly human. **A friendly smile can do more for healing sometimes than a mighty drug.** *There are people who, just by their affability, help others to understand their problems and their conditions such that healing begins to take place immediately. In order to be affable,* **we must stretch ourselves past where we want to be and allow ourselves to feel what the patient is looking for and needs.**

ABILITY. When you get right down to it, unless we have the training and the ability to do our job, the first two A's do not amount to very much. In order to be a good physician in today's world, we need to really know the tools we learned in medical school and in our training programs and be able to use them in a healing manner. **Our abilities as physicians are essential to the whole process of healing.** *If an orthopedic surgeon doesn't know how to work with bones,* *it doesn't matter a great deal how accessible or how affable he (or she) is.* **Mother Teresa said it like this**: *"The biggest disease today is not leprosy or tuberculosis, but rather the feeling of being unwanted, uncared for and deserted by everybody. The greatest evil is the lack of love and charity, the terrible indifference towards one's neighbor who lives at the road side assaulted by exploitation, corruption, poverty and disease." So, it seems to me that this triad of the three A's is an excellent model for a holistic physician and their office staff.* **We need to meet people where they are, work with them at the level** *they* **can understand and allow ourselves to be involved** in-depth *in the healing process with them. Using the three A's can bring about a clearer understanding of how to function as holistic physicians and give to those who need it a* true *experience of healing.*

Again, when I was president of the AHMA, the message I wrote in the November/December 1983 news- letter addressed this very point, and I will also quote it in its entirety, as it also is no longer in print.

In the September 1983 issue of Continuing Education, *I found an article which was stimulating and exciting to me. It triggered a response which I think needs to be spoken to and expressed. The title was: "The Singular Sadness of Numerical Madness," and it was written by Richard B. Lee, MD. The thrust of the article was this: somehow,* **with our technology and our ability to pull statistics together, we have lost sight of the individual patient.** *He makes the point that, if we do not have statistical significance to work* *with, the importance of a single case history is lost and even labeled "anecdotal." This point has long been a problem that I have wanted to address. Most of the work I have done has been with individual cases, and my reporting has been on my clinical observations and the results of the work I have done when partnering with patients on their healing journey. This approach has been labeled "anecdotal" and therefore insignificant, as well as of no value.*

*To me, it has seemed that a case history is just that—a case history. Each person in my office with a problem was asking for help, and each one considered the statistical significance of a certain disease cure rate to be relatively unimportant. I am not downplaying the importance of statistics with my point of view. I think statistics have their value. However, to me, statistics occur more like background music in a play, which is not meant to be the primary focus of our attention during the play. In other words, **we must not get so wrapped up in statistics that we cannot see the importance of dealing with an** individual **patient who has his or her own** unique **accumulation of symptoms**. When this happens, the patient is left without any real help, having nowhere to turn and no one to depend on to get that help.*

Biblical literature is replete with information about the importance of the individual. Jesus talked about the Good Shepherd who left the 99 and sought after the one lost sheep. He talked about the woman who had a special place in the *kingdom of heaven because she contributed her widow's mite. It has been said: **if there is ONE white crow, it proves that all crows are not black.**[62] It is not the masses who have changed the world. Rather, **it is the individual person here and there who has done the most to change the world** —the Jesus, the Buddha, the Mohammed, the Paracelsus, the Mother Teresa—the individual person who was in tune enough with his or her spirit that s/he was able to kindle Light and Life in the lives of other people. This kind of contribution does not arise from the masses. It happens because the Spirit of God illumines one soul here and another one there.*

***Mother Teresa** worked with the masses of people in India; however, she **did not see individuals as diseases or people without faces. She saw them as individual beings with a soul and a spirit that needed to be awakened.** In looking at research in our organization [AHMA], it is nice to have some statistics to work with, but I pray that we never lose sight of the fact that **a** true **physician works with patients as** individuals **who are created in the image of God;** and, in reality, each one of us is striving to know ourselves, to be ourselves, yet one with God.[63] That is what healing is all about, isn't it?*

When I am **face-to-face with someone** in my office or addressing the reality of the microcosm (my patient) within the macrocosm (the

---

[62] www.goodreads>quotes>527170-if-you-wish-to-upset-the-law-that-all-crows-are-black (William James).

[63] Cayce, Edgar. A Search for God – Book 1, 1942 (reprinted 1970, 2018), Chapter 2.

world around us), then that one individual in that moment becomes truly a great mystery to me, and **nothing in the world is as important or as exciting.** It does not matter whether s/he is young or old, black, white or brown-skinned, "curable" or "incurable"—each patient is unique and wonderfully different.

Diseases can be the same. Therapies can be the same. No two patients though **are** *ever* **the same.** *Statistics are important when we treat diseases and use therapies, and they fall into the background (as they should) when we work* uniquely *with* each *individual patient.* The "bottom line" message then is this: **if I, as a physician, bring my training and my caring into the picture and can** *truly* **connect with the seeking part of another** *unique* **individual,** at that point a marvelous thing happens. **On some level, within** *both* **of our beings, healing takes place. This unique healing experience is truly** *far* **more important than the curing of any one disease.** Consequently, *it is the individual patient's involvement in his or her own healing process that becomes* the *critical component* of laying a *solid* foundation for our Living Medicine home.

My frustration early on in the practice of medicine consisted primarily of patients who were *not* taking responsibility for their healing or even their health conditions. I am delighted to say that this experience changed dramatically for me through the years once I learned to *give a patient's body back to its rightful owner!* By doing that, more and more of my patients started to become aware of how important lifestyle changes, thought processes, living conditions and environmental factors impacted their well-being. They also began to look at the part *they* play in their own health and well-being. This paradigm shift was very gratifying to me and reduced my frustration with practicing medicine significantly.

I truly believe that *we need to be much more aware of and focused on the physician/patient partnership* and the way in which everything we do creates who and what we are. **Whatever we** *think* **manifests in what is going on in our lives and in our bodies.** What our emotions are in relationship to things that happen in our lives can be worked with in many ways, including body work, bio-feedback, exercise, nutrition and electromagnetic field therapies.

Working with the symbols associated with the endocrine glands in our dreams can also be very helpful. The impact of prayer and meditation on the whole healing process has now been validated[64] and can become part of a person's healing armamentarium. We need to **be less focused on killing diseases and more focused on enhancing the immune system and allowing people to engage in their own healing process.** We need to work with music and color, beauty and touch, as well as joy and laughter as important therapeutic tools.

Through the research done by the amazing neuroscientist Candace Pert, PhD[65] (1946-2013), we now understand that **molecular structure can change with emotional impact**. She scientifically puts into context the reality that **cells have consciousness** and that **a relationship exists between thoughts, emotions and the actual cellular structure of our body.** *Her work* is pivotal in helping us to establish and fortify a solid foundation for our home of Living Medicine, because it *integrates the science and art of medicine in a very usable way.* In a similar, though different, way, Larry Dossey, MD's research[66] demonstrating the **"non-local" healing power of prayer** shows us that this tool **is likewise a mighty healing force**.

Creating a solid and stable foundation for our house of Living Medicine is *ongoing* work and a difficult process; *and*, like any living process or living body, it **requires that *all* aspects of the foundation be integrated and work well together**. The concept that best explains this idea is the same one that Dr. Ann uses to explain how OMT works: *tensegrity* (see diagram[67] and explanation below), the engineering principle that was used to build the geodesic dome. The

---

[64] www.ncbi.nlm.nih.gov>pmc3396089.

[65] Pert, Candace B, PhD. Molecules of Emotion: The Science Behind Mind-Body Medicine, 1997.

[66] Dossey, Larry, MD. Recovering the Soul: A Scientific and Spiritual Search, 1989.

[67] McCombs, Ann, DO. Text written by Dr. Ann and original artwork commissioned by her, ©1994.

German engineer Walther Bauersfeld (1879-1859) was the inventor of this structure, which was later developed by Buckminster Fuller (1895-1983). This principle allows a system to maintain integrity and stability by always being in a state of *balanced tension*.

To illustrate: *if you touch the many-sided ball* (made up of wooden sticks and elastic cord) in the diagram below *at any point, every other point on the ball moves also*, to some extent. This is how the *fascia* (connective tissue) of the human body also works. Because *every* muscle, nerve, organ, bone, etc. is surrounded by this strong, shiny, thin covering. *We are connected by this fascia, head to toe.* Were it not for this fascial envelope that surrounds *all* parts of us, we would not be able to be upright human beings, much less people who can move with grace and ease.

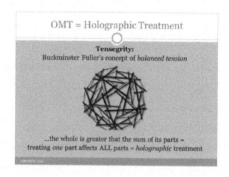

Tensegrity is also the concept that illustrates why physicians and dentists "can no longer be separated in today's healthcare environment, especially given that **approximately eighty percent of many chronic disease states today are directly or indirectly caused by dental interventions**[68] (amalgam fillings, root canals, surgical extractions left to heal by secondary intention, electro-galvanism, orthodontic treatment that leaves the bite in a poor occlusal relationship relative to the whole body, etc.). The 'Americanization' of medicine separated these specialties so significantly that *physicians and dentists must now work together* in order to treat these problems *successfully*, be-

---

[68] Strong, Gary A. DDS. Does Mercury From Dental Amalgams Influence Systemic Health? and 34 other references – see www.icnr.com>uam>hgcourse>Reading.

cause the structure and function of the mouth is so interrelated with the structure and function of the whole body." [69] As a DO who has been working side-by-side with a DDS since 1990 to create *optimal* health for herself as well as her patients, Dr. Ann's opinion is that bodies can never have the chance to *fully* heal unless they have a *stable foundation* upon which *to* heal. If the body is not *balanced from head to toe*, which may include "all things structural" (e.g. *functional* jaw orthopedic appliances and *dynamic* pedal orthotics) along with *all* forms of OMT to bring about this "balanced tension" explained by the tensegrity model, it will always be compensating. It will never feel "right" or calm internally (at peace within itself) without this kind of balance. Individual physicians or dentists can diagnose the causes of chronic illness. However, in Dr. Ann's experience, it takes a physician *and* a dentist working *directly* together to provide the necessary support for patients to even have an *opportunity* to heal from a state of chronic disease. To facilitate a deeper understanding of how physicians and dentists can accomplish this task, the Holistic Dental Association[70] was formed in 1978, followed by the International Academy of Oral Medicine and Toxicology[71] in 1984 and the American Academy of Biological Dentistry in 1985, which became the International Academy of Biological Dentistry and Medicine[72] in 2005. Just like "it takes a village to raise a child,"[73] it also takes a *collaborative team* of health care providers to bring about *optimal* health and *true* healing.

Another example of what it takes to create a solid *and* stable foundation requiring *all* aspects to be integrated and work well together occurred when the AHMA was formed in 1978. "Strength through diver-

---

[69] McCombs, Ann, DO and Riniker, LaVar, DDS. "The Physician-Dentist Team: Optimal Health for the 21st Century," Holistic Medicine (AHMA journal) and HDA Communicator (Holistic Dental Association journal), Spring 1997. This article can most easily be found currently on Dr. Ann's website: www.nonprotocolmedicine.com.

[70] www.holisticdental.org.

[71] www.iaomt.org.

[72] www.iabdm.org.

[73] "It Takes A Village To Determine The Origins Of An African Proverb" www.npr.org>goatsandsoda>2016/07/30.

sity" was listed among the first in our list of goals and objectives. This goal meant "to provide a common ground where diverse interests in medicine can find unity in ideals and values, recognizing the diverse approaches that converge on a unified philosophy of holistic medicine." Clearly, as we soon discovered, *this goal was a process* that was easier said than done, which is best illustrated with the following analogy.

We have all had the privilege of listening to a symphony in which the individual instruments *together* provide a harmonic sound that stirs us to our very depths. We could easily take any *individual* instrument and listen to it with appreciation and then listen to another one with added appreciation. However, it is not until the sounds of each instrument are *combined* that what is experienced becomes music that touches the soul. If each instrument were to play a different tune, all would be confusion and discord. However, when all the instruments in a symphony are *united in a single purpose* to produce a singular piece of music, the result often reflects great artistry that touches the soul and can move us to tears.

In the field of Living Medicine, we have physicians (MD's, DO's, ND's, DC's) of all types and specialties: general practitioners, family physicians, neurologists, urologists, surgeons, oncologists, obstetricians, pediatricians and the list goes on and on, as well as many types of other health care providers (homeopaths, acupuncturists, dentists, etc.). Some physicians are teachers and professors, others are researchers or consultants. Dr. Ann recently showed me a book outlining many *nonclinical* careers for physicians.[74]

Regardless of what any of us choose to do with our medical training, as Living Medicine physicians, we are all still in service to people whose souls inhabit a human body. The Apostle Paul said it this way in I Corinthians, 12:18 (bold is mine): "But as it is, God arranged the organs in the body, each one of them as He chose. If all were a single organ, where would the body be? As it is, there are many parts, yet one body."

So, **what is it then that makes Living Medicine different?** As I see it, the difference lies in the fact that **we are *unified in our desire to be of service* to each *person with whom we come in contact*,**

---

[74] Stacy, Sylvie MD, MPH. 50 Nonclinical Careers for Physicians, 2020.

keeping the values of the unity of body, mind and spirit in the *foreground* in our work with patients, independent of whatever approach we may be utilizing in our individual specialties. If this is our goal (or our ideal), it follows logically and sequentially that, **as we do the work we need to do, *we ourselves grow* and *then* stimulate growth within others.** Because we are not afraid to address the *spiritual* nature of our being and open ourselves up to guidance from the "Power That Is Greater Than Ourselves," we can expect to be involved in *a healing process that is* truly *transformational.*

If we as physicians are actively working *together* with patients towards a single ideal, it makes no difference how many diverse approaches or philosophies we have. We might even be diametrically opposed to a specific therapeutic approach. However, *if our purpose is the same, the result will be like the harmony we hear in the beauty of a symphony.* The **strength** that **comes from diversity** is likewise multi-dimensional and can be tremendously beautiful, *and* transformational. Life is never easy, and the *living* process has its own ability to make us stretch and grow.

Years ago, I sat on a speaker's platform with a Japanese man who made an important statement. He said:*"Hard jobs* are done by those who can. *Impossible jobs* are done by those who care. *Transforming jobs* are done by those who are committed."* Notice that he never mentioned *easy* jobs.

We, *as physicians*, do not have an easy job to do. It is a hard one, a very hard one. Yet *we can do it because we are capable.* We are well-trained, and we are good doctors. We know how to treat sick people, as well as those who are already healthy, and we are learning more about how to do our jobs every day. We can work in hospitals and in emergency rooms. We can work in the backwoods, in farm communities and in big cities. Because we are *not* locked into rigid structures from the past, we are willing to open our minds to the healing techniques that come from the past *as well as* the present.

We have a *wonderfully* hard job to do...*and* we can do it! Because we care, we can do an *impossible* job. Not only do *we* care, our patients and people in general care. They care about each other, and they care about us. When we have a *transformational* job to do, we do it because we are committed. *We are bound to a standard of excellence that brings research and science in medicine forward into their proper place with the* art *of medicine*, transforming the field of *medicine* into what it **really** *is: an art, with science as its tool.*

Truly great artists, like the **truly great physicians**, are those who go beyond the techniques that they use well and tap into the transforming essence of the Spirit. They **lose themselves as ego structures** (like the captain of the battleship finally had to do to avoid hitting the lighthouse!) **and connect with the Source of all Life through creativity.** As we work with the concept that "my spirit beareth witness with thy spirit" (Romans 8:16) and, as we work with healing others, *we* also have the *opportunity* to be *truly* healed. Jesus said: "I have come not to destroy the law, but to fulfill it" (Matthew 5:17). We have come not to destroy medicine, but to awaken it to the knowledge and reality that, as Edgar Cayce said: "**all healing comes from the One source,**"[75] **whether it be the knife, castor oil or a prayer.** We are *trained* to bring about cures, though we are *dedicated* to healing. We are *trained* in the *science* of medicine, though we are *dedicated* to the *art* of medicine.

As we use the *art* of medicine to transform the whole field of medicine, *we* can also truly become transformed. The belief that patients should be informed and can make wise decisions *for themselves* provides the foundation for the possibility of *true* healing to happen for *all* of us. This statement makes great sense to me, though I have also learned, in the words of Stephen Covey[76], "*common sense isn't always common practice*," especially for those of us on the pioneer path.

The true essence of Living Medicine is healing from the inside out. This principle takes the concept of holistic medicine (which deals with the healing of the body, mind *and* spirit) to a whole new

---

[75] www.edgarcayce.org. Reading 2696-1.
[76] Covey, Stephen. The 7 Habits of Highly Effective People, 1989.

level, as the following words from Ezra Taft Benson quoted by Stephen Covey[77] emphasize so clearly and paraphrased by Dr. Ann:

[Spirit] *works from the inside out. The world works from the outside in. The world would take people out of the slums.* [Spirit] *takes the slums out of people, and then they take themselves out of the slums. The world would mold* [people] *by changing their environment.* [Spirit] *changes* [people], *who then change their environment. The world would shape human behavior, but* [Spirit] *can change human nature.*

This principle also reflects the poignant lesson that The Quota Club and I learned in a very graphic way when I practiced in Wellsville, Ohio in the 1950's (see my recounting of that story in the playroom chapter), and *it is one of* the *fundamental principles of Living Medicine.*

The emphasis in **Living Medicine** clearly **focuses on Life and the *living* process, so that the disease can be incorporated into the Life process as a *living* thing.** As a patient *lives* their life, a disease can become a *part* of who and what they are, without *focusing* on the disease, by just simply allowing it to be *a part of* their growth. When I speak to other physicians, I recognize that the Physician Within me contacts the Physician Within the other doctor. **We must work *together* to bring LIFE back into the heart of medicine. *The Physician Within and the Physician Without* are part and parcel of the whole and *provide the bedrock* to create a SOLID *and* STABLE** foundation for our house of Living Medicine.

---

[77] Ibid.

3

The Living Room

The front yard and the front door represent our *conscious* mind. As we open our front door to others and invite guests into our living room, we and they step into the part of our home where *real life* starts to take place *on a conscious level*. This is where relationships begin, where our own *living* process interacts with the *living* processes of others who come in and out of our home, and where we recognize our connection to other people. Our living room is what truly expresses or manifests to others how we see *ourselves*, so that we can relate to them.

As we take our first breath upon entering our living room, we can become aware of the air that we breathe in our Living Medicine dwelling place: it is the very energy of Life itself. We cannot live without it. For this gift of Life we feel grateful, recognizing that **one of the most fundamental principles of Living Medicine is gratitude**. This principle was squarely brought to my attention when my daughter (Analea) and I had lectured together in Minnesota. When people came up to talk to us after the lecture, someone asked me: *"What's your secret to life?"* I was trying to come up with a cute response yet was unable to find the right words, at which point Analea gave me the elbow-in-the-ribs treatment and said: "Oh, you do so know the secret, Mom. You *dwell in gratitude*." I said: "Oh, yes, you're right!" And then someone asked me: *"What is the difference between being grateful and dwelling in gratitude?"* My response was: "If I am grateful for something, it's because I have received something from the *outside* of me, brought into my dwelling place, either by myself or others. I am either grateful for it or not. If I receive it with gratitude and incorporate it into my life and my being, it becomes mine. If I choose *not* to be grateful for that gift, I can get rid of it or do something else with it, and it does not become part of my being. To *dwell* in gratitude is different. It's the way I live, it's the way I think, and it has become so much a part of my personal being that, like air, I can't live without it." So, for me, gratitude is one of the fundamental essentials of our Living Medicine dwelling place, in addition to Life itself. This Living Medicine principle can be illustrated with the following story from an article I wrote[78] (excerpted below) which, ironically, very much applies to our current experience of "sheltering in place" during the COVID-19 pandemic of 2020.

> *I had a friend, James, who moved into a retire-*
> *ment home at age 89. It was a nice, though*
> *small, room set up with the things he really*
> *needed. He had traveled, lived in many coun-*
> *tries and had just auctioned off his home,*
> *which contained his precious art objects and*
> *the best of everything. Once, when I visited*
> *him in his new home, he told me that he was*
> *so happy. He loved his upstairs room, where*
> *he could look out over the rooftops. He had a*
> *little plant in the window that he cherished. All*
> *his needs were being taken care of. He said:*
>
> *"There's even that magic box." He went over*
> *to the thermostat and said: "See, it is magic. It*
> *is hot in the room right now; but, if I push this*
> *lever down, it cools off. If I get too cool, I push*

---

[78] McGarey, Gladys Taylor, MD. "Facing Hard Times Gracefully," *Venture Inward: The Magazine of the A.R.E. and the Edgar Cayce Foundation*, March-April 2009.

the lever up, and it gets just the right amount of heat. It's a magic box." I was so delighted with his comment. The ability to turn a simple thermostat into a magic box that takes care of your environment is pure genius and reflected to me the very essence of this Living Medicine principle: James was dwelling in gratitude.

In our world today, where everything is shifting and many of us are having a hard time adjusting to all the changes, it is our challenge to reframe our lives and start really appreciating what we do have and stop focusing on what we don't have. In his long life, James learned what my mother called "making do."

As children in India, my siblings and I learned to entertain ourselves by taking what was available and using it for whatever we were imagining or working with. My sister and I learned to knit by finding pieces of wire and sharpening them down to make knitting needles. Any piece of yarn or wool that we found we would wrap into balls of yarn and knit clothing for our dolls. Our Ayah (the name for nanny, nursemaid or "other mother" in India) *had shown us the basic knitting stitches, and we improvised and learned how to adjust those stitches to make doll clothes. When Life's circumstances cause us to cut back to our basic needs, we often find we are happier and more content. Life gives us choices regarding what is really important and what brings us closer in tune with our ideal. We can moan and groan about the economy and the hardships that come our way, or we can dwell in gratitude for what we do have. This moves us out of fear and into the flow of Life and allows us to see magic in the simplest of things.*

Next, we need to really look at the furnishings in our living room, the pictures on the walls and the general ambiance of the room, which define our individual personality. If we do not pay attention to these things, and if *we* do not know who and what *we* are, then our neighbors and friends may never have the opportunity to get to know us for who and what we *truly* are. As we get to know *ourselves*, we can begin to *love* ourselves, which allows others to truly love *us*.

Through the years, I have introduced myself by saying: "I'm Gladys McGarey. I'm a physician." A few years back, after I had said that to somebody, I stopped and thought about that statement. I am a physician. What happens if I *lose my license* to practice or find myself in a position where I can *no longer* practice? In 2000, at the age of 80, I *voluntarily* gave up my medical license when "managed care" became the norm in *conventional* medicine. To me, **"managed care" is the *antithesis* of Living Medicine**. I then wondered: *was I no longer relevant without my medical license?* Absolutely not! I *still* introduce myself in the same way I always have, because I came into this world *knowing* I was going to be a physician. I then *became* a physician, I am *still* a physician and I will *die* as a physician because *it is my life purpose*. The same can be said for *everyone*, no matter what their profession or career choice (artists, teachers, parents, etc.), when that profession or career is in harmony with one's life purpose. My profession helps to describe the *work* that I do in the world, it colors *everything* that I do, and I view the world around me through that lens; yet it does *not* reflect my *whole* identity. Stephen Covey[79] said: "life is a mission and not a career," and we both agree with this statement for those whose life purpose is in harmony with their life's work.

---

[79] Covey, Stephen. The 7 Habits of Highly Effective People, 1989.

I once had a patient in my office who had been given the diagnosis of multiple sclerosis (MS). She came in very excited, because she had a dream to share. In her dream, she saw a little girl about four years old lying face down in the mud. She picked her up, turned her around and looked into the little girl's face. Much to her surprise, it was her own face. She held the little girl tightly and said: "Oh, I love you! I really, really love you!" When she awakened and shared the dream with her husband, he said: "Yeah, well, okay." "NO! NO!" she said: "You do not get it. I really, really love that little girl." This woman grew up being taught that loving oneself was wrong. She was supposed to love *others*, but not herself. She grew up believing that loving oneself was selfish and self-centered. In her dream, and in the waking state since that dream, she knew she loved this little girl, and that it was right. She felt stronger and more at peace when she accepted the message that loving herself was good. Her body language, as she was talking to me about what had happened to her as a result of her dream, was much more loving and powerful than I had ever seen on her previous visits to my office. She was in the process of reclaiming her power through learning to love herself, realizing that doing so was really *not* self-centered *or* selfish at all!

Many of my patients through the years, particularly women, have had trouble accepting and loving themselves, or even caring for themselves. It is easier for them to deal with other people's problems and needs that are more in line with what they have been taught is "God's will." They were raised to focus their energies outside of themselves. However, this is *not* what Jesus taught. The central core of His teaching is: "love the Lord, thy God" and "love your neighbor as yourself " (Matthew 22:34-40), much like the Lord's Prayer reminds us to forgive *our* debts as we forgive our debtors (Matthew 6:5-15). We also talk about *unconditional* love, yet one of the conditions we put on ourselves is that we must be *worthy* of loving ourselves. We know our own faults better than anyone else, so we judge ourselves to be unlovable. *Love really needs to be without judgment or conditions,* which is how God loves *us*, and how we can learn to love ourselves *and* one another.

One of the ways that we can learn about unconditional love is from animals, some of whom are our own pets, who, for the most part, love us *no matter what*. These animals can also be quite intuitive. This is one of the main reasons Dr. Ann has had a "therapy dog" in her medical practice since 1992. She has often observed these sentient beings be able to "break the ice" and soften the hardest of hearts of some of her more challenging patients, causing them to be more open and receptive to healing when her therapy dog was present than when he wasn't. Sometimes, it is *only* these amazing therapy animals that can bring enough safety and comfort to veterans with PTSD to help them heal from their painful experiences. Dr. Ann has also had some personal experiences with both horses and dolphins that created profound "aha" healing moments for her. Much research has already been done to show the therapeutic value of "animal-assisted therapy" across many healing professions, as well as in the classroom.[80, 81]

Our family had just moved to Phoenix when my four-and-a-half-year-old son (Bob) came running into the house and said: "Mama, I know if I make a friend, and he makes a friend, and he makes a friend, and he makes a friend, it'll go all around the world and come back to me." Somehow, he knew it had to start with *him*. Wouldn't it be great if that philosophy permeated *all* our lives!

If we do not take care of ourselves, we cannot take care of other people. A good example of this is what happens every time you get on an airplane. The flight attendants always give a little sermon before the flight begins. They say: "If the oxygen mask drops down in front of you, *don't* put it on the person next to you before you put it on yourself." In other words, you cannot take care of the person next to you, if you do not take care of yourself *first*. Another example is a woman who, when she is pregnant, must *first* care for herself—

---

[80] www.icaad.com>resources>the>benefits>of>pet>therapy.

[81] www.uclahealth.org>animal>assisted>therapy>research.

mentally, physically and spiritually. As she does this, she nurtures the child growing within her.

It remains evident all through our lives that **a central part of our service to one another is, *first and foremost*, an internal process of *self*-care, then taking what we have learned into the outer world**. However, for many of us, it is harder to receive than to give. *To truly receive, we must accept the fact that we are in need.* This is often difficult to do, because accepting help reminds us of our vulnerability, our humanness. The good news is that, when we live fully in our humanness, we are not only healthy *within*, we also have greater gifts to give to *others*. **When we admit our need, we are empowered to receive.** As we receive help from others, we are filled. Then, we can give more fully of ourselves to others.

Another aspect of self-care is learning that to be lovable we must be "love-able." *To be able to love, we must start with loving ourselves, which is not being selfish, it is being self-aware. It is not being self-centered, it is a higher form of self-care.* As we seek peace and love for this world, we must start with ourselves and learn, as my patient with MS did, to "really, really love" that little girl or little boy within. This is a lesson I had to be reminded of again during my recovery from a total hip replacement. I was going through the process of allowing my body to heal, allowing myself to accept help from family and friends and being forced to focus on my own healing process from within. *It was a blessing to me to open my heart and receive the love and healing that was sent my way.* It was a reminder of so many lessons I have shared with patients. My twelve-year-old grandson brought me the series of books he had been reading. As I healed, I allowed myself to be twelve years old again and enjoy that growing aspect of myself.

The concept of *knowing ourselves* is fundamental to Living Medicine. *True* healing occurs when patients take responsibility for and begin to understand who and what they are, what their emotions are, how they feel about things, as well as how they respond to changes in their lives. They must decide whether they want to keep the windows closed and the blinds down, or whether they are willing to open the windows wide and let the light shine in. We must know what we want in our living room, our *true* dwelling place, where we get to tell *our own* story and share it with others. This principle was never made clearer to me than when I spent three months in Afghanistan in 2005 hearing the life stories of individual women.

Thirty women from ten different villages in the remotest part of the Bamiyan District gathered together in the "living room" of a house where we held a week-long conference for mothers. Initially, we had to get permission from the *men* who were leaders in these villages *prior to* even considering the possibility of working with their women. At first, the men objected, saying they did not want their women away from their homes. They feared what their women would be exposed to, as women in Afghanistan are not permitted to move freely outside of their homes. When we explained that we wanted to talk to their mothers-in-law *instead of* their wives and daughters, they agreed for reasons we really did not understand.

We wanted to meet with these women because they had had babies and stories to share that had never been told. *No one had ever listened to them* because their stories were not considered important. As we sat around on the floor in this "living room" woman-to-woman and told our stories, *the living essence of healing could be felt the whole time.* What we learned from this gathering is presented later in this book. The experience brought out their pain, their joy, their fears and their hopes, as they shared their pregnancy histories with us. As the women communicated with *each other*, it helped *us* understand more about the life issues, challenges and illnesses they faced.

I have a physician friend who describes illness as "social communication"—a socially acceptable way of letting ourselves and those around us know that something is not quite right, or that something needs to be repositioned or removed. In our Living Medicine dwelling place, there may be an old couch that is of no further use and ready to be tossed, just as in the living body there are times when certain parts are no longer serviceable and need to be surgically removed. The following story illustrates this concept perfectly.

I had a patient in my office who really needed surgery and *really* did not want it. In trying to convince him to have this lifesaving surgery, I suggested he might try to think of it more like a gardener pruning a tree. The purpose for cutting off the limbs is not to punish the limbs or to kill them. Instead, removing the part that no longer serves the tree harnesses its energy to grow more vigorously and completely. Pruning focuses and directs the Life Force to bring more life and health to the tree as it grows to fulfill its purpose. My patient then told me he could now understand why I wanted him to have this surgery, *because he* was *a gardener* (which he had not previously shared with me). He was then able to move forward with his surgery without resistance.

Jesus said (paraphrased): "I came to give you Life [so that you can] have it more abundantly" (John 10:10). It is this abundant life that we are seeking for our patients *and* ourselves in Living Medicine. **Living Medicine includes the reality of pain and sickness, depression, anger, the sense of failure and even death.** However, **it** *also* **includes joy, laughter, hope, love and the breath of Life.** The living room is where we allow *all* our senses into our dwelling place. *By awakening* all *our senses, we will see more clearly, hear more deeply and feel more surely.* To reach the mountaintop, we must first cross the valleys. If we are afraid to allow ourselves to feel grief and pain, we cannot feel the fullness of joy and happiness. **Happiness does not exist by itself without sorrow, fear or conflict.** It occurs by working through the difficult times and finding our way *through* them, instead just trying to "get over" them. It also means, "in part at least...the fruit of the desire and ability to **sacrifice what we want** *now* **for what we want** *eventually*," according to Stephen Covey[82] (italics are mine). These valleys of emotion *will* enter our house of Living Medicine at some point in time, and it is our challenge to *accept* them, *experience* them and *do something positive* with them, which can sometimes be a real sacrifice in the moment!

---

[82] Covey, Stephen. The 7 Habits of Highly Effective People, 1989.

It is in our living room where we can enjoy music and entertainment according to what we choose. If we choose to listen to a symphony, we must understand that *each* musician as an individual, needs to understand their music, their instrument and the composition that s/he is working with. *Each musician* will spend hours upon hours practicing and perfecting his/her skill. In a symphony, even the musician who plays the triangle must understand his instrument, the place where his note will be played and the proper way in which to do this. In the overall rendition of the symphony, that note played by the triangle may seem insignificant; yet, without it, the symphony would not be complete. When I think of the discipline, the patience and the concentration required for a musician to play that *one* note, it is truly awesome. Likewise, the flute solo is also important; however, without the harmony of the *rest* of the orchestra, it would not have such a powerful impact. In an orchestra, *every* note played by *every* musician is important for the *overall* beauty of the rendition. So, it is with the human body. **There is no part of our body that can be complete without the cooperation and harmony of *all* the other parts.** Every molecule of our physical body is in relationship with every other molecule. Every story told in the living room becomes part of the "music" of our Living Medicine home, helping us create a *truly* harmonious *living* space.

During his training as a resident in ophthalmology, my youngest son (David) had a professor who, when David presented a case describing the patient's life and other aspects of his health, said: "I don't want to hear about any of that. All I want to hear about is the eye." Granted, the eye needs to be studied and understood as a single structure. However, *by itself*, it is useless to the person. **Everything that happens to a person, is *recorded* in their physical, mental, emotional and spiritual "bodies."** We are *a work in process*, and are *constantly* creating who and what we are, even at one hundred years *young*! We are even creating our past, moment by moment. Every thought and every emotion that I experience is as much a part of me as the food I eat. The thoughts I think, the words I say, the books I read, the pictures I see, the nature I adore—*all of these* make up who and what I am. *The more I understand the instrument that I am, the more I practice focusing on my ideal, so that my thoughts are constructive and healing.* As a result, my instrument will be truer in its presentation of the musical note that I am in this lifetime, *including my role as a physician.*

Many living rooms have a fireplace as a focal point, and I find its symbolism quite fascinating. I was talking with friends a while ago about fireplaces and chimneys and was reminiscing about the fireplaces where I grew up in India, as well as the three hearths in the Phoenix home where my children were raised. We only used the one in the living room, and it became a true centerpiece for gatherings. We all enjoyed building the fire, stoking it and keeping it going on winter nights. We watched the flames, talked about the colors and fantasized about what was going on within the fireplace. Once in a while, something would happen—the damper would get stuck or there would be an obstruction in the chimney—so that the airflow would stop, with smoke building up and filling the room. The fire itself would smolder and sometimes die, unless we got the airflow moving properly again. In the meantime, we would suffer from burning eyes, an inability to see well in the room, coughing, irritation of our lungs and just general discomfort. The fire, if contained and properly mixed with oxygen, was a joyful and healing family experience. However, left uncontrolled, the fire became an irritating and even dangerous experience. Occasionally, one of the children would put too much wood or flammable material in the fireplace, and we had to wet it down to control it.

If we take the symbol of the fire in the fireplace and apply it to ourselves, we can see the importance of **the proper control of energy** as it moves up from the *third chakra* (where anger, fear, resentment and hate reside, manifesting as *fire*) to the *fourth chakra* or the love center, where *air* is the element of healing and love. We know that *anger can cause many destructive forces within the entire body, just like fire can, if uncontrolled.* However, when the Life Force energy moves up through the chimney as fire carrying any of the emotions associated with the third chakra, we find that the force of *Love lifts and transforms these emotions into beauty and calmness.* Fire is energy, air is energy and emotions are energy, as is love, *and* all *living energy is creative, because it is a* living *process.* **Energy needs to flow or move**, so that the fire, or the creative energy at the level of the adrenals, can truly be an active force. If the oxygen does not mix with the fire adequately, the flames smolder and die. In dealing with ourselves and our children, *if we keep telling ourselves we must not get angry, we can either make that creative energy smolder and die, or build up and become explosive.*

Recognizing, acknowledging and validating emotions is essential to our growth, just as controlled fire is essential to life. Many of our chronic illnesses result from *misdirected* energy. For example, "anger gone blind" can result in a *feeling* of hate as either a *short-term emotion* (e.g. "I hate vegetables") or a *long-term sentiment* (e.g. teenagers who "hate" their parents all during their adolescence). It can also result in an *action* like rage (e.g. verbal and/or emotional abuse) or, in extreme cases, violence (e.g. physical abuse).[83] If misdirected or suppressed, these emotions can result in arthritis, high blood pressure, stomach ulcers, colitis, dermatitis and other conditions.[84] **Medications can often control the** *symptoms* of these illnesses; however, **until the proper flow of energy is re-established,** *true* **healing cannot take place.** We seem to understand anger when it explodes and causes trouble, just as when a fire burns out of control, yet we have trouble understanding the smoldering anger that creates the conditions for the explosion. *Anger can be held in our bodies* for years *before it explodes as illness.* If we depend completely on medications to control the symptoms, the smoldering fire continues to pose a problem. However, when we allow this energy to flow again through

---

[83] Fischer, A. et.al. "Why We Hate" (research article), 2018. See www.journals.sagepub.com>emotion>review>why>we>hate or https://doi.org/10.1177/1754073917751229.

[84] https://www.fatherly.com>health>risks>of>holding>in>emotions

prayer, meditation and the use of the "fruits of the Spirit,"[85] then *true* healing can take place. *Anger in and of itself is* not *bad*, and we all have times when it erupts. Even Jesus chased the moneychangers out of the temple in anger. *Anger itself is a clear emotion*, with many ways of being expressed *without* causing harm to ourselves or anyone else. We can go dig in the garden, we can go for a run or work out at the gym or we can find some humor in the situation. Perhaps we should recognize anger as someone visiting us in our living room and *choose* how we are going to treat that particular person: will we engage them in conversation, ignore them or rebuff them?

Every day we face experiences that come to our front door requiring us to choose what we will do with them and how we will relate to them. Most of these decisions are made on an *unconscious* level, while other decisions are reached consciously. Each experience that comes to our front door can appear in the form of people, ideas, activities in the outer world, changes in our environment or anything else that we might experience, day by day and moment by moment. As we open our front door to these particular experiences, we either allow them to step over the threshold *or* we send them away. If they do step over our threshold, we then have the choice to stand in the foyer, talk to them for a few minutes, then let them go *or* invite them in, perhaps for a cup of tea and a social time together, and then let them go. We may even invite them in for dinner and then decide to have them stay overnight—sometimes for a day, sometimes for a week, sometimes for months and maybe even for a lifetime.

If, when opening our front door to the emotions of fear or anger we simply let it go, we will probably not even remember the situation. If the experience is appealing enough to invite these emotions in for whatever length of time we choose, then our involvement with them as part of our actual dwelling place becomes stronger. If we allow the fear or anger to enter and stay with us for months or even years, it

---

[85] The nine attributes of a person or community living in accord with the Holy Spirit, per Galatians, Chapter 5: love, joy, peace, patience, kindness, goodness, faithfulness, gentleness and self-control.

will bring its relatives of envy, jealousy and self-pity. As these relatives become stronger and invite in *other* guests, the very essence of our being, our soul, gets pushed farther and farther into the part of our dwelling place that moves us into a mode of survival. The soul's ideal then becomes tucked away in its office, where it continues to do its work and perform its duties. It presents a façade to the outer world that everything is just fine. The soul's ideal even convinces itself that things are adequate. However, the person's self-image, self-worth and *inner* reality will be so overwhelmed by the presence of anger within its dwelling place that the soul hardly recognizes itself. The outer world might even label the individual as "an angry person."

This concept reminds me of an amaryllis bulb given to me one Christmas that bloomed and graced my home. Then the flower wilted, with the leaves drying up and the bulb shrinking down, until it looked totally dead. Thinking there was no life left, I put it out in my garden and forgot about it. I imagine that the bulb felt useless, abandoned and unloved. As a part of Life that appeared to be no longer alive, it *felt* dead. However, it landed in a part of my garden where the soil was rich with Life. A rain shower came along, the sun came out and *it* began to feel a stirring, an awakening within itself. *It* somehow knew it was *not* dead. Within its very being, its Life Force and its ideal (life purpose) were *still* present. Somehow, *it* knew that it could be, and should be, revived. *It* knew that it had to reconnect with the Life Force within its roots in order to penetrate the earth and move the ground apart, so that it could begin to recreate itself and build a *new* dwelling place, as it is doing right now in my garden, in order to be able to bloom again.

In observing the life journey of that little amaryllis bulb, I learned that **Life is *always* reaching for Life, even after *what appears to be* death**. Dr. Ann and I both have also seen this principle manifest when *some* people who are in the process of dying reach for the Life that is coming to *greet* them in death. For me, this principle was demonstrated when my sister (Margaret) was dying and she announced to the family gathered around her: "Ayah is here." Dr. Ann experienced the reality of this principle as her mother was in the dying process following her third stroke. Amazingly, she squeezed Dr. Ann's hand *with the hand that had been affected by her stroke*, then opened *both* eyes (not just the one *un*affected by the stroke), looked up and smiled *at the exact same moment* that Dr. Ann felt her deceased father's presence in the room. The agitation her mother was exhibiting just prior to this event *immediately* resolved without her having to be medicated for it. She waited for Dr. Ann's brother to arrive, then died early the next morning while she and her brother were both sleeping in her room (during "the only ten minutes" Dr. Ann had slept the entire night), an event that is quite common among the dying.[86]

When we choose a profession, it comes to our front door as a welcome guest. If we take it in and allow it to take over our *whole* life, however, so that the very essence of our being is squeezed into a small corner, we may lose contact with who we really are. There may come a time when we can re-awaken to the *core essence* of our being (our soul) and commit to transforming our professional obsession (or whatever the issue is) and reclaim our dwelling place as well and our life. Or there may be times when we literally are so shrunken within ourselves that we find ourselves being tossed out. Like Esau in the Bible (Genesis 25: 29-34) and in the 1963 Italian film[87], we "sold [our] birthright [the right to be recognized as firstborn] for a mess [meal] of pottage [lentil stew]."[88] Basically, Esau sold his soul for a fleeting pleasure. This can happen to *any* of us who have been shortsighted and gotten our priorities confused. The beautiful thing is that *it is never too late to reclaim our birthright.* Once we recognize our situation, we can always *make a different choice,* and with God's help, rebuild. At that point, in order to continue living, we have the option to create an *entirely new* dwelling place. This *new life* and new dwelling place can be more beautiful, more serviceable and more in tune with the world around us and our own nature than the old dwelling place ever was.

---

[86] www.dyingmatters.org>page>spiritual>aspects>of>death.

[87] www.en.m.wikipedia.org>Jacob_and_Esau_film.

[88] www.en.m.wikipedia.org>Mess_of_pottage

This kind of paradigm shift is also what is happening right now in the field of medicine. **The *true* spirit of healing and the *art* of healing have been so neglected and so misunderstood that it requires a new structure.** This awareness was driven home to me recently when I was listening to a lecture given by an artist. My interest was captured by a statement this artist made: "Through art, we find our humanity." I think that statement would have had greater impact and been more accurate if it had been said as follows: "*through **ALL** of the arts*, we find our *true* humanity," as it is through the arts that we are able to tap into our *true* creative nature and move ourselves towards our life purpose (our ideal). To reach the goal of reclaiming our *true* humanity, we need to build a solid and stable foundation that will hold the *structure* of Living Medicine. In so doing, the *entire* human race will have the opportunity to evolve into the True Human or Divine Human. This latter process involves the "the Word [becoming] flesh" (John 1:14)—the One, the I AM, the all-inclusive, *uni-dimensional* form—taking on a physical body to become a *two-dimensional* form (a spiritual being dwelling in a physical body). Transforming the soul's two-dimensional form into its *unique and individual three-dimensional*, body-mind-and-spirit form (the True Human or Divine Human) involves the discovery and manifestation of one's life purpose (ideal) and bringing that ideal into alignment with the planet's purpose (ideal). Edgar Cayce's term for this evolutionary development of the human race is "the fifth root race,"[89] which is discussed at length in the summer 2020 edition of *Venture Inward.*[90] Paula Polcini describes this evolutionary process in detail in her book,[91] inspired by her experiences with her bi-polar son-in-law (Max). She likens this journey of the human soul to that of the chambered nautilus, which consists of gradually enlarging compartments. "As the little creature that lived inside the shell outgrew one chamber, it moved on to the next, where it could grow and develop

---

[89] www.edgarcayce.org. Readings 470-35 and 5748-6.
[90] Venture Inward: The Magazine of the A.R.E. and the Edgar Cayce Foundation, Summer 2020.
[91] Polcini, Paula. PM: Man's Journey from Darkness to Light, 2013.

further." (Interestingly, Polcini points out that the human body is literally made of building blocks whose proportional ratios always equal PHI [1.618], or the ratio of *each* of the chambered nautilus' spiral's diameter to the next spiral. As a result, she concludes that PHI must be the ultimate expression of Divine Proportion!) Polcini then goes on to state: "Man is the only creature with consciousness....Each man is responsible for his own development to leave [his or her] low-vaulted past to build more stately mansions, 'til thou at length art free, leaving thine outgrown shell by Life's unresting sea!' (Dr. Oliver Wendell Holmes)." These concepts are "heady stuff," as Dr. Ann would say, yet oh-so-important to help we physicians *truly* understand *our* life journey as well as the *healing* journey of those we have taken the Hippocratic oath to serve.

As physicians we can find *our* truth and be healed through medicine, especially by practicing the *art* of medicine, so that we can then become *true* facilitators for the healing of others. With the tremendous advances the *science* of medicine has made, we need to allow those advances to remain in their proper place and perform the work that *they* need to do. However, **we must not let science take over and displace the *real* heart and soul of the work of healing—the *art* of medicine—which, together, we call the PRACTICE of medicine.**

To illustrate these points, let me tell you about a patient I saw many years ago. She had severe dermatitis on both arms. We worked together for some time, trying to find a solution. I finally sent her to a dermatologist. When she came back to me, I realized that there was something going on inside of her which probably was not going to get fixed from the outside. The Physician Within *each* of us needed to take charge at this point. I said to her: "I would like you to start visualizing a field which has been burned. The ground is black because it has suffered from a grass fire. Then, the rains come and, here and there, little green sprouts of grass begin to show through the blackened dirt. As you continue to watch this field, you begin to see more green shoots coming up. Do you think you can do this?" She began smiling and said: "Yes, I can. I'm a retired firefighter." Somehow, through the work that we had done together, **the Physician Within *me* and the Physician Within *her* made contact and came up with the *right* solution for *her.*** Together, we were able to remove the blockage of energy within her that was obstructing the flow of life and her healing. **By using both the *science*** (seeing the dermatologist for a thorough work-up) **and the *art* of medicine** (the visualization I had asked her to do), **she was able to heal.**

One of the manifestations of the fruits of the Spirit that is so vital in removing the blocks to our energy flow is *forgiveness*— forgiveness of ourselves and of others. The importance of this principle was taught to me many years ago when my grandson, David, was about six years old. We were sitting around my dining room table with my grandchildren playing the game "I see something green or red (or whatever)," and the other children then had to guess what it was. The game went on for a while, until David looked at me and said: "You know, I never give up." So, we played for a while longer. Suddenly, he jumped off the chair and started running around my living room; running around, running around and running around. When he climbed back up on the chair, he looked at me and said: "I never give up – but, sometimes, I take a rest."

I was so pleased with David's response, because it was a very important lesson for me as I worked with patients who had chronic illnesses. These patients would work with their therapeutic modalities for long periods of time and then become weary, knowing that they could use a rest; yet, if they took a rest, they would feel guilty. They might go to a birthday party and have a piece of cake, which was not on their diet, and their guilty feeling for doing so would make the problem worse. If, however, they were able to say to themselves: "I'm not giving up, I just need to take a rest," their healing would continue. **The messages that the body gets from the mind are *vital* to the healing process**. When the body understands that taking a rest is not only an *acceptable* thing to do, that it is the *right* thing to do, healing continues.

The central part of the Lord's Prayer (Matthew 6:9-14) states: "Forgive us our debts as we forgive our debtors." It then goes on to say: "Deliver us from evil." Perhaps evil could be viewed, in this context, as illness. One definition of evil in the dictionary is "harmful or injurious," and another is "accompanied by misfortune or suffering." Used in these contexts, illness becomes something that we would like to be delivered from. Illness sometimes leads to death, and the word *evil* spelled backwards is *live*. *Whether we truly overcome an illness or just learn to live with it, we are asking in this prayer for Divine help in addressing it.*

Laughter offers us another way of moving our energy. Norman Cousins (longtime editor of the *Saturday Review*) scientifically demonstrated this through his work in the mid-1960's, which is described in detail in his book.[92] Edgar Cayce said that Jesus was even able to joke on the way to his crucifixion. Then, perhaps, using Jesus as an example, we can truly access healing energy, even in the form of laughter. **No matter what modality is used in the healing process, as *we* are healed, so is the world around us healed.**

Our living room offers a place where we can feel strong emotions and, sometimes, even destructive ones. These can resemble fearsome storms. However, when these storms clear, we often find new hope, cleaner air and an opportunity to rebuild. If we give ourselves the chance to *experience* these storms and *live through* them, then take the time to *rebuild* from them, things can become significantly better, and we often *feel* stronger.

Strong emotions can represent such storms. For example, if we think thoughts of hatred, those thoughts become part of us. However, *if we* feel *angry and express it "cleanly" and without malice, those thoughts do not become a part of us...they simply dissipate.* I once heard a preacher say that, if we *immediately* start looking for answers when faced with a choice on how we respond to a situation, then someone has to be right and someone has to be wrong. The emotion of anger may then quickly take hold and can turn into a short-term

---

[92] Cousins, Norman. Anatomy of an Illness: As Perceived by the Patient, 1979.

emotion or long-term sentiment of hatred, as previously discussed. If, on the other hand, we respond in a logical manner, taking into consideration *all* aspects of the situation, *even if we are feeling angry*, then hatred is *not* the motivating force—reason and rational thinking are. The choice we can *then* make can be a *conscious* one that creates *unity* instead of divisiveness.

Another illustration of this preacher's principle can be understood when we distinguish *the difference between arguing and discussing*. In an argument, almost always someone must be right, and someone must be wrong. *Arguments* are usually also very personal and can become quite passionate and emotional. *In a discussion*, however, we are working with *facts*, which are *not* personal, and we are in control of our emotions. *Anyone can learn to argue. Learning the art of discussion, however, is a real and valuable skill.* In distinguishing these two behaviors, we can then see how *even* the *simple, mundane choices* we make in *every* moment of our daily lives then *become significant*, as they are *either leading us* towards *our life purpose (our ideal) or* away *from it*. When an individual becomes aware of his or her life purpose, their choices can then become like "second nature" to make, moving them closer and closer to their ideal. In this same way, a person can learn that *emotions (even strong ones) are feelings one can have, express and then release,* instead of *becoming* those feelings and having their actions be constantly ruled by them. In this way, a person can redefine him or herself as just *a person with strong emotions*, instead of thinking of themselves (and others thinking of them) as "an angry person."

One final, personal story also illustrates these principles. From the time I was a small child, I hated my hands. In my mind, they were huge and ugly, partly because of being red, swollen and bleeding from the chilblains—painful, itchy swelling of the skin with repeated exposure to extreme cold. I had this condition in the fall of every year at boarding school, where there was no central heating system. I especially hated my hands when compared to my sister Margaret's hands, which were slender with long, beautiful fingers. I was so embarrassed by my hands that I actually sat on them as much as I could. My feelings of hatred towards my hands did not change until I was a senior medical student and observed a female surgical resident scrubbing in for surgery who had hands that were *even bigger* than mine! *Instantly* I realized that her hands were just one of her *tools* to help her become the surgeon she wanted to be. From that "aha" moment on, I stopped hating the hands that were helping *me* to become the physician *I* wanted to be (my ideal). My feelings of hatred for them then transformed into total gratitude, and I even started wearing rings!

Our living room can also provide a safe place to heal from pain, whether it is physical, mental, emotional or spiritual in nature. **There is healing energy in pain.** *Physical* pain gives a signal, informing us of where we might have a problem that needs addressing. It is felt at the physical level unless it is interrupted by nerve damage, or we are anesthetized, asleep or under the influence of hypnosis or drugs. While *physical* pain itself does not always suggest a problem, it still **needs to be felt and acknowledged.**

Mental and *emotional* pain also needs to be felt and acknowledged. If we do not allow ourselves to experience these pains, we may not be sensitive to or aware of what is happening in our lives. We may move into senility, Alzheimer's disease or some form of psychosis. With *spiritual* pain—if we try to avoid it—we shut ourselves off from other people, the world and God. We actually die within ourselves. If we really allow ourselves to feel pain on *all* levels, without getting stuck in it, but rather just **recognize it and try to understand the reason for its presence and its message**, we are then able to alleviate it *or* make peace with it, so that we can truly live a full and abundant life.

Another emotion we will encounter in this room of Living Medicine is fear. *Fear needs to be recognized for what it is and dealt with.* The following patient's story illustrates this point well.

This woman called me because she was scheduled to receive a blood transfusion and was afraid to do it, because of her concerns about AIDS and hepatitis. She had undergone chemotherapy for lung cancer and her blood count had dropped dangerously low, requiring the need for a blood transfusion. It seemed a little strange that she was afraid of AIDS and hepatitis when the illness she was struggling with was already so devastating. However, her fear was present and *very* real to her, so I had no reason to question her feelings. I explained that there were millions of people who had transfusions without contracting an infection. In addition, the current rigorous checks and safeguards ensured that the chances of contracting AIDS or hepatitis from a blood transfusion remained very, very slim. *This did not alleviate her fear.* Finally, we discussed the possibility of her looking at her fear in a different way: perhaps she could realize that, somewhere in this world, there was a person who loved and cared for her enough to give her their very life's blood so she could live. This individual did not know who she was, and she had no knowledge about that person, either. This act represents *true* unconditional love, from one heart to another. One must give and the other must receive. Perhaps the healing and love in the blood would offer exactly what she needed for the chemotherapy to become more effective. If she accepted the blood transfusion as a gift of love, hope and faith, without fear and doubt, it could present the miracle she was looking for. Just to visualize those loving red cells going through her body, touching all her cells with love and healing, bringing the physical gift of oxygen to all parts of her body, would be a creative and loving thing to do. From this perspective, she was able to go ahead and get the transfusion. **Seeing** the **possibility** of the life-giving energy of that blood transfusion, Living Medicine became a reality in her life.

Another guest we will find in our living room is *grief* and her close cousin, *depression.* Currently, Mother Earth is expressing Her grief via the tsunamis, the hurricanes, the earthquakes, the floods, the landslides—and the COVID-19 pandemic that has been manifesting all around the world. We have not listened to what She has been trying to tell us. *We are bleeding Her by removing oil from the very heart of Her being.* This oil represents *Her* life blood and cannot be replaced. We have no transfusion to offer Her. By removing Her minerals, we are causing Her osteoporosis, manifesting as sink holes and other structural disasters. *None of these minerals can be replaced.* In our ignorance, we are doing to Her what our ancestors did to President George Washington: to help him heal, they told him he needed a bloodletting which, of course, is what killed him.[93]

Mother Nature bestows upon us many sources of energy. We have solar energy, hydrogen energy, wind energy and energy from water—resources available to us *that are renewable and sustainable* due to their ability to constantly replace themselves. I wonder when we are going to invite Mother Nature into our living room and say: "We love You, we want to work with You, and we want to keep supporting You in any way we can." She has been so hospitable to us, yet we have been so rude to Her. She has welcomed us at every level and accommodated us as best She could. We have not only ignored Her, we have *brutalized* Her. We are so afraid of what Mother Nature can do that we attack Her and try to control Her every chance we get, to further *our own* wishes and wants. Knowing that Mother Nature is in such deep pain, I like to visualize taking Her in my arms, sitting in a rocking chair and rocking Her like I would one of my children or grandchildren.

This idea became very personal and real for me when I celebrated my seventy-fifth birthday with my daughter and her two sons. Daniel (the older boy) said to me, "Nanni, how old are you?" I said: "Daniel, I'm seventy-five years old." He said: "Is that old?" I replied: "Some people think it's old, but I don't try to wipe the wrinkles off my face. They belong there, and I deserve every one of them." He then said to me: "When you get to be really, really old and you are really, really sick, I'm going to pick you up in my arms and take you up to your room and rock you, and rock you, and rock you." *That was the nicest birthday present he could have ever given me.* I knew that he had a little book that talked about this. The important thing, though, is that

---

[93]   https://www.pbs/newshour/health/dec-14-1799-excruciating-final-hours-president-george-washington.

he remembered it. Now, if we could just transpose that experience to Mother Earth—who *is* really, really old and really, really sick—and just "rock her and rock her and rock her," how much healing could come about, how much loving could be manifested and how truly grateful She would be! *Mother Earth* never asks for anything. Paraphrasing the celebrated poet Hafiz: and "even after all this time, [*Her*] Sun [has] never [said] to [Her] '**You owe me**.'" [94] If only *humans* could be such grateful stewards of *Her* energy! She would certainly be a welcome guest in my living room at *any* time.

During the Gulf War, I had patients who came to see me for depression. There were so many of them complaining of depression that I began to wonder: "Why now? Why are people going through more depression now and more than they had been several months before?" I began asking people when their depression started and what it was like. As we looked deeper at what they were dealing with, what emerged was that *they were all grieving*—for a son or a relative who was overseas, for the people in the Middle East who were suffering, and for Mother Earth, whose oil fields were being burned. Most importantly, they were grieving for themselves; and it was a deep, *soul-level grief*. We realized it was *not* depression, and that **there is a significant difference between grief and depression**. After the shock of 9/11 in 2001 and the fear associated with it, this phenomenon occurred again. Currently, we are *still* at war in the Middle East (and now, in 2020, we are *also* in a different kind of *world* war in the form of a global pandemic) and grief *still* poses a serious problem.

I looked up grief and depression in the dictionary and found that these words are not even synonymous. The synonyms for ***grief*** include *suffering, sorrow, regret, disappointment* and *distress*. The synonyms for ***depression*** are *rejection, gloom* and *downcast*. Even in the dictionary, these two emotions are not considered the same. Yet, **in our culture, we deal with them as if they were identical issues**.

---

[94] Paraphrased in part from an original poem by Ladinsky, Daniel. The Gift: Poems by Hafiz, 1999 (p.34) inspired by the spirit of Hafiz in a dream.

As I began working with people who learned to express and address their grief, their whole feeling of sadness shifted. They realized they were *not* depressed—they were simply grieving. *Grief is an emotion, an experience that we all share.* There are times of grief in everybody's life, and that emotion is completely personal and individual. What one person grieves over might not be something that another person finds sad. I have patients grieving over a cat or a plant that died, a job that has been lost or a remark that someone made that caused them to lose their self-respect or relationship with that particular person. Grief is an ongoing emotional process that we all deal with in our own way, day by day. *As we recognize our grief and work through it, allowing ourselves to grieve, we grow.* If we try to suppress it or bypass it, it can become a deep-seated problem that may manifest as an actual *physical* symptom. In my opinion, **grief should *not* be medicated; it must be *experienced*. Depression, on the other hand, can be a *medical* condition** that sometimes even runs in families. **It should be identified and dealt with by a medical professional,** in case medications (pharmaceutical or natural), other modalities (e.g. special forms of counseling) or, sometimes, even Divine intervention are needed to treat it. *To confuse grief with depression,* however, *does not allow for the* normal *process of growth that is part of our lives as human beings.*

This aspect of life was brought to my attention by a patient/friend whose husband of thirty-eight years died and she, of course, was grieving very deeply. After two years, she came into the office one day saying she did not know what was wrong with her. She was still grieving her loss, and people were telling her it was about time she "got over it." My response was that **we do not have the right to tell another person when the grief process is complete. How long it takes, the form it takes and how it is dealt with are completely *individual* processes and part of the growth of *that specific soul.*** We just need to support each other through it.

The scripture passage from John 11:35 speaks of when Jesus was called to the grave of Lazarus, who had been dead for four days: "Jesus wept." In John 11:36, the Jews said: "Behold, how He loved him." **Love and grief are very close companions.** If we love someone deeply, there are times when we are going to grieve. If we *truly* care about the world around us, there may also be times when we might find ourselves grieving for the suffering of our world. In my own life, I have experienced all kinds of grief. For example, when my daughter (Analea) died, I experienced a very painful and deep grief, probably because *she* was ready to leave this world and *I* was not ready to let her go. When my sister Margaret died, though, my experience of grief was entirely different. The following thoughts have helped me understand the difference between these two experiences of grief when it entered my living room.

Some of the happiest people I know are those who allow themselves to grieve. They are individuals who seem to be able to tap into the deep, profound emotion of love that touches their deep core, recognizing a "love that surpasses all understanding" (Ephesians 3:19). When something happens in their life that is painful, they allow themselves to *fully* grieve…then they go on with their lives. I watched my sister Margaret do this when she moved into a retirement home, and I had the experience of being able to grieve in this same way when Margaret died. The following article, [95] reprinted and updated below, is a perfect illustration of how this kind of grief can occur and be dealt with when experienced and understood in the context of a person's life.

> *Margaret was my sister. She was there when I was born, and I always knew that her loving spirit was with me, no matter what was going on. Her calm and tender love was as real to me as my own breathing, and it still is, though on March 8, 2017 she graciously moved into the next chapter of her soul. I was deeply sad.*

---

[95] McGarey, Gladys Taylor, MD. "God's Other Door," Venture Inward: The Magazine of the A.R.E. and the Edgar Cayce Foundation, October-December 2014.

My grief was tempered, however, by the reality of her loving life, the impact of which still shines beautifully in my own life.

Margaret lived her 99 years fully, with all of Life's good times and hard times, and she was grateful for them all. In our family, she was always the calm and peaceful one who prayed daily for each one of us. One of my nephews, when he was going through a difficult time, said: "I'll get through this, because I know Aunt Margaret is praying for me." Margaret lived by herself after her husband died until she was 96, when she moved into a retirement home across the street from her church. She was healthy and doing well when she moved in there. It was fun for her, because all the residents there were aware that they were going to be in this home until they died. In filling out the form for the move, there was a question about whether she played a musical instrument. She wrote: "drums." This was because, when we were girls in India, our Ayah taught her to play the Dholak (an Indian drum played with both hands). Her retirement home had a harmonica band, and she became part of it.

In the spring before she died, I was talking to her on the phone when she asked: "Do you remember Betty?" I had just spent a week with Margaret, and I remembered Betty well. Margaret continued: "We were going to go to a wedding, and I was supposed to drive, but Betty up and died, so I had to drive by myself." She was sorry about that, and this was her way of saying she expected it, because this was just the reality of saying what was so and moving on.

While I was visiting her, Margaret wanted us to have our picture taken together for the retirement center. When that was done, she sat up straight and said: "Now it's time for the obituary picture." Seeing my surprise, she said: "That's what we do around here."

Once Margaret told me about two of her lady friends who called each other every day to check in. One day, one of the ladies called the other lady several times throughout the day and got no answer until late afternoon. When her friend finally answered the phone, she said: "Oh good, I thought you had died," to which her friend responded: "Not today."

Like Margaret, these wonderful women lived full, fruitful and loving lives—and they were not afraid of death. They accepted it as part of Life, with both grace and peace.

Margaret was sick for only two weeks, in and out of the hospital, before she died. She was moved into hospice care when it became obvious that she was ready to move on. All her children and grandchildren were able to spend time with her. Her youngest son and his wife were with her at the end, as she drifted in and out of consciousness. She began singing hymns, quietly at first, then her voice got strong, and she began singing Indian hymns known as Bhajans. Every so often, she would stop and say: "Ayah is here." She sang for two hours! Her minister came and spent a short time with her, said a prayer and a blessing, and, before the minister was out of the room, Margaret took her last breath. I glory in the sight of her being welcomed by a multitude of the Heavenly Hosts as she, accompanied by our Ayah, sang and drummed their way to her "reward." Her son and his wife wished they had recorded the singing. However, they were in such awe and bliss that they had to live it and tell us about it later, so we could, each in our own way, experience the blessed glory of such a passing!

Both Margaret and Ayah welcomed me into this world, and I know they will be there when I am ready to make my journey out of it. Their presence is still very real to me every day of my life. I am really sad that Margaret died. However, my grief was short-lived, because I had the opportunity to watch this amazing woman live her life until the moment she died. I knew that she was ready to go, which made it easier for me, with love, to let her go. She was such a shining example for me of **"aging into health,"** the natural process of just breathing until you don't breathe, embracing Life fully and engaging with it in every moment, until it is done. That's why I feel that Margaret's passing was really a celebration of her life.

Grief is natural and needs to be expressed. It helps to share grief with other people, while allowing it to manifest as it will. One of the best ways of working with grief is to *reach out to someone else who is grieving*. As we share our grief and our love, we *each* become stronger, and the world becomes better for it. *When lonely people retreat into their aloneness, they become engulfed in it*. However, if they look around for another lonely person, they may find the courage to break out of *their* aloneness. When we are at war (whether in reality or in a pandemic crisis like COVID-19 in 2020) and the people all around us are grieving, Mother Nature is also grieving, and the *world* is deeply, deeply caught up in grief. At this particular time, it becomes *essential* that we recognize this UNIVERSAL GRIEF and *reach out to see what we can do to help each other*. In doing so, hope and joy and Life itself can move and not remain blocked by *unacknowledged* grief. We can say: "That's so sad," and then *move toward helping each other* carry our respective loads, working *together* to create a more loving, more compassionate and more considerate world. The *deepest* grief, however, is when we feel *separated from our Source*, or God. Bringing God back into our lives comes about when we recognize that grief and have the courage to deal with it.

One of the universal laws is *"like attracts like."* When we choose to have a home—whether "home" is our body or the actual house where we live—it is a place where we can manifest our desires, our hopes and our dreams. The key for us is to recognize these hopes, desires and dreams and accept them when they show up at our front door. For some reason, in *our* culture, we have created the myth that desire is an evil thing. Yet, *creativity is derived from desire*. Put into action with imagination, desire allows us to create and develop new concepts and new ideas. Somehow, we have condemned desire by associating it with the Garden of Eden story in which Eve saw the fruit and found it desirable. When and why desire became evil from that point on is a mystery to me. *Without desire, we would never move out of our stuck places*. We really would not grow.

Desire leads us to the possibility of experiencing our great human potential. What we desire then becomes *our choice.* If we choose beauty, health and joy in our lives, we attract those things into our lives. This does not mean the circumstances that arrive are necessarily beautiful or joyful. *Our* response *to the circumstances that we have attracted results from our desires.* On the other hand, if our desires are constantly negated by thoughts of our own inadequacies, or if we judge or punish ourselves for having our desires, then the desires that may produce beautiful results are averted or destroyed. For example, if I desire an abundant life that is healthy, I need to accept the *aspects that create health*—diet, exercise, positive thoughts and harmonious relationships—things which bring health into my life. Otherwise, my *negative thoughts*—my anger, jealousy or frustration—*attract negativity,* which grows and becomes more powerful.

This principle was manifested in my life one Christmas when I went to visit my youngest son in Flagstaff, Arizona. His five-year-old son met me at the front door and opened it without saying a word. He looked me up and down several times. Finally, looking at me straight in the face, he said: "Nanni, you're a good person." To me, that was the most wonderful Christmas gift he could have given me. I came into the family's living room and was accepted not just as their mother and grandmother, I was also accepted as a "good person."

What we accept into our living room is our choice. Usually, it is an invited guest. Sometimes we have someone show up at our front door whom we did *not* invite. How we receive that person is our choice. When we open the door and let someone into our living room, *that act impacts our whole life.* In this house of Living Medicine, there are certain experiences that come to our front door. For the most part, we either allow and welcome them in, *or* we close the door and do not allow them to enter. A *third option* also exists: sometimes those experiences are literally foisted upon us, and we have absolutely *no* control over allowing them to come in. In these instances, we feel as if we have *no choice* at all. However, because of Victor Frankl's (1905-

1997) book[96] detailing his experiences as a prisoner in *four* Nazi concentration camps during WW II, losing both parents, his brother and his pregnant wife in the process, we learn that we *still* have a choice, even under the direst of circumstances. In his words: *"When we are no longer able to change a situation, we are challenged to change ourselves."* In Covey's words, the principle exhibited by this remarkable man is this (bold and italics are mine): "In the midst of the most degrading circumstances imaginable, Frankl used the human endowment of *self-awareness* to discover a fundamental principle about the nature of [humankind]—***between stimulus and response, [a person] has the freedom to choose.***"[97] As a result of the unwanted and unwelcome experiences that showed up at Frankl's front door, he discovered that when we as humans cannot avoid suffering, we *can still* choose how to *cope* with it, find *meaning* in it and *move forward* with renewed purpose. Covey would say that Frankl did this by choosing to become responsible—*"response-able"*—by taking as much control of his circumstances as possible with his *ability to choose his response* to them. Frankl did this by identifying a purpose in life that he could feel positive about while imprisoned, and then he immersed himself in imagining that outcome. As a neurologist and psychiatrist, he later developed a theory from his experiences that he called *logotherapy* (from the Greek word *logos* or "meaning"). Frankl came to understand, through his experiences as a prisoner of war, that **the primary drive of human beings is** *not* pleasure, as Freud maintained; rather, it is **the discovery and pursuit of what we personally find meaningful**. *The importance of identifying one's life purpose cannot be underestimated*, which is addressed throughout this book and was discussed in detail earlier in this chapter.

In my own life, this concept became very real to me some years ago when I was going through an extremely difficult time. There were experiences and feelings that, over a period of years, kept presenting themselves at my front door. During those times, I was neither strong

---

[96] Frankl, Victor, MD. Man's Search for Meaning, 1946.
[97] Covey, Stephen. The 7 Habits of Highly Effective People, 1989.

enough nor in a state of consciousness where I could welcome those experiences and feelings into my home. I could not have handled the impact of those issues on my life when they came knocking at those times, and I was certainly not ready to deal with what they would have done to my entire life back then. So, I turned them away for many years. Finally, different things occurred in my life such that *my front door was literally blown open when my husband of forty-six years asked me for a divorce.* These issues then entered into my living room in such a way that I could not turn them away, and I could not get rid of them. *My life has not been the same since.* In many respects, it has been *richer* in spite of the fact that, metaphorically speaking, all of the furniture in my living room had to be changed or updated.

Somebody once asked me how I was able to manage what was going on in my life during those years. As I thought about it, I thought about how a desert tree roots itself. If it hits a caliche layer, which is comprised of clay so solid that it resembles cement, it has two options. One option is to let its roots grow out sideways, without attempting to penetrate the caliche layer, in which case it dies. The other option is for it to put all its energy into breaking through that caliche layer until it reaches its Source, at which point nothing can knock it over. The winds of time and the storms that hit do not affect it, because it remains solidly connected to its Source. I feel that, through the years, even though I was not dealing *directly* with those issues at the time, I *was* in the process of putting my roots down deeply enough until I reached *my* Source. In the past, I had focused all my energy on maintaining my home and taking care of my patients. That way of life fit with my ideal or life purpose, which was to serve God with all my heart, mind and soul. I had to let my taproot be in direct contact with my Source, or God, in order to do that. As a result, I believe that when my front door was unexpectedly blown open, *that Source is what gave me the strength to go on with my life.* Presented with a new opportunity to grow, I chose to move on by redecorating my home. I *could have* sat down in my rocking chair and let Life pass me by. I am thankful that I was able instead to feel the excitement of the *new* situation that has so enriched my life since then.

There are so many things in Life that come to our front door which, when we welcome them, make life more wonderful. One of these is the value that *human touch*[98] has in the very act of survival.

This was brought to my attention recently when I heard a preacher tell the story of a grandfather whose daughter had a very premature baby girl. Weighing just a little over a pound, she remained in a hospital incubator. Since the infant's father was not in the picture, the nurse asked the grandfather if he would assume the role of her father when he went to see his new granddaughter. This would mean coming to see the baby every day, talking to her and telling her that he loved her. When he did so, he was to touch her with his fingertips and massage her little hands, feet and body with his fingertips. The nurse said: "This baby will connect your voice with your touch, and that is going to mean as much to her as anything that we can do here." The grandfather happily agreed to do this, and *the baby thrived.*

Two other examples of the importance of touch come to mind. One occurred during World War II, where some children in a London orphanage were held and touched while others were not, despite receiving the same care. *The ones who were not touched deteriorated, those who were touched, thrived.*[99] The second example is from a television program I remember seeing years ago called *Omni,*[100] which focused on touch. It showed a person who was given the job of watching people use a pay telephone. This individual would go up to the person who had been talking on the phone and say: "You know, I really need to make a phone call, but I don't have a dime. Could you lend me one?" (This was when phone calls cost a dime when made from a pay telephone booth!) *The people whose arms he touched*

---

[98] https://www.khca.org>files>8>reasons>why>we>need>human>touch>more>than>ever.

[99] https://theconversation.com>infancy>and>early>childhood>matter>so>much>because>of>attachment.

[100] www.omnitv.ca.

when making the request all gave him the dime. If he did *not* touch their arms, they did not give him the money.

In *conventional* medicine, many physicians never touch their patients unless they use their stethoscopes.[101] In my experience, *many people really hunger for a friendly touch.*[102] We get jostled and bumped around in crowds. However, **to be touched by a person who cares and who is interested in us can be very, very therapeutic.**[103] As we have learned and have seen from the "me too" Movement,[104] *inappropriate* **touching can cause lifelong damage and** *must* **be acknowledged and addressed for** *true* **healing to become possible.**

I have found that an *appropriate* hug will frequently not only help to relax a patient, it can also start the healing process.[105] Many people who would really love a hug are afraid to initiate it. This reluctance may be due to fear of rejection and, in part, because they may have never initiated personal contact. It is difficult for them to get past their fears and shyness, and they feel that initiating a hug would be inappropriate. The comment "*To be lovable, one must be love-able,*" speaks to physical touch. *To be touchable, we have to be "touch-able."* To me, this means that if we are hungering for a touch, we should be looking for those people who seem to need a touch and ask them if we can give *them* a hug.

During one of the live-in programs at our clinic in the mid-1980's, a group of participants gathered for healing at a soul level. There were fifteen people in the group, and all of them were very self-contained, self-sufficient people who really did not want *any* physical contact with another person, much less a hug. As we went through the ten-day program, they had dreams and experiences that helped them to identify the underlying feelings that were keeping them separated from each other. One of the participants was an elegant, sophisticated,

---

[101] www.theconversation.com>touch>creates>a>healing>bond>in>health>care.

[102] https://www.healthline.com>health>what>is>touch>starvation.

[103] www.greatergood.berkeley.edu>hands>on>research>the>science>of>touch.

[104] www.MeTooMVMT.org.

[105] https://www.healthline.com>health>why>you>should>get>and>give>more>hugs

self-contained woman in her early forties who felt that she and her twin sister never really wanted to hug or touch each other, even as little girls. Several people even made the comment that they had always felt like lepers who were shunned and never touched because of their disease. By the end of the program, *every one* of the participants had come to grips with their feelings of possibly having spent a past lifetime as a leper in which they had been ostracized and were not allowed to touch or be touched. As they accepted and understood this possibility, their feelings began to change and, by the end of the program, they experienced no problem with hugging and touching! They even were able to sit at the table close together and hold hands during grace.

I believe that the importance of touch represents one of the reasons physicians recommend massages.[106] Of course, massage also is important for lymphatic drainage, as well as to stimulate the nerves, to help coordinate the cranial-sacral and autonomic nervous systems and to alleviate muscle spasms. On a deeper level, though, massage is vital because we, as human beings, need to touch each other and to be touched by one another in a loving, caring, helpful way. *Inappropriate touching is neither loving nor caring—it is selfish and crude.* In a world such as ours, to have the negative aspect of touch eliminate the positive is to let darkness overtake light. As we get older, it is very important that we give and receive love and caring in the form of touch. In fact, *this world needs a program in which small children and the elderly can interact.* The little ones need to experience the loving touch and wisdom of a time-worn hand, while the elderly need to encounter the smooth, soft touch and pure energy of a toddler. This concept had been a dream of Elisabeth Kübler-Ross, MD who was a friend and patient of mine for many years. Elisabeth loved tea parties. No matter how sick she was, she would offer me a cup of tea in her living room; the place in *her* home where people first gathered for tea parties and discussion groups.

---

[106] www.health.harvard.edu>the>healing>power>of>touch.

Ever since 1957, I have had a weekly Edgar Cayce study group in my living room, where we discuss all manner of topics dealing with our spiritual growth. So, this area of my home also represents my sanctuary and holy place. This is where many tears have been shed as well as much joy and laughter. It is where my grandchildren come and pull out the pillows and spend the night. It is very much a place of ongoing Life and experience.

The way we greet people who come to our front door depends on what is going on in our lives. There are times when a person comes to my front door and says: "I'm so happy to see you. You haven't changed a bit." I may not have seen them for ten years! While this is meant as a compliment and I take it as such, the more I think about that, I am not so sure it *is* a compliment! *If ten years have gone by and I have not changed, should I consider that a compliment?* Perhaps it reflects that my life has stood still, and I have not really learned a lot or experienced my living process at a deeper level. I do not need to look the same as I did when I was sixty or seventy years old. I would hope that some of the things I have experienced would show on my face and person, so that my experiences can help my children and grandchildren benefit from them. My little grandson, Taylor, is a true teacher of this principle, as the following story illustrates.

We were discussing things of interest to a six-year-old boy one hot Arizona day in my living room when, suddenly, out of the clear blue sky, he stopped all conversation. Looking me straight in the eye, he said: "Nanni, I think the meanest thing that anybody could do would be to kill all the teddy bears and the blankies." I thought that was really cute, and we went on talking about other interesting subjects to him. When I thought about it later, I realized that Taylor's statement wasn't just cute, it was very profound and insightful. Our *children have so much wisdom to share with us,* and it is so easy for us to think that our thoughts and deliberations are more important than their insights. I agree with Dr. John Trainer who said: **"Children are *not* a distraction from more important work—they are the MOST important**

work"[107] To me, Taylor's idea of killing the teddy bears and blankies says that we need to be very aware of the nurturing aspect of Divine energy, and that we cannot live life *fully* without letting tenderness and compassion enter into our everyday lives. We have done so much harm by taking away the arts and other nurturing programs from our schoolchildren in our attempt to have them fit into certain proscribed patterns. I wonder what the children in war-torn Iraq are doing for teddy bears and blankies. No wonder the world is angry. Perhaps we could have a project of dropping teddy bears and blankies instead of bombs. Maybe we cannot give them the material teddy bears and blankies, however, we can all pray for them and hold them in our hearts with our loving concern. Now I realize that it is not just the little children who need this kind of concern, ***the child in each one of us is looking for and wants and needs to share love and compassion.*** This realization was never clearer to me than when a young person I know was entering medical school and told me he had taken his blankie with him. It is pretty much of a rag by now, though it continues to offer him comfort. I believe that, because of his awareness of his own needs, he will become a truly great doctor.

In the Bible, when Jesus and his disciples were faced with the problem of feeding five thousand hungry people, it was a small boy who produced the five loaves and two fish that Jesus blessed and used to feed them all, with twelve baskets left over (John 6:1-14). We all need to look for and accept the gifts children bring to us, and then bless them and share them with each other, because, let's face it: Life is not easy! Mary Poppins' statement "A spoonful of sugar makes the medicine go down" truly represents a fundamental truth. **We *all* need some sweetness and tenderness in our lives, especially to help us deal with the "medicine" we *all* must take in Life.** We *all* have some difficult karmic patterns to live with. As we recognize these patterns in ourselves and others, we can look for opportunities to be kind and gentle with the hurt parts of ourselves and others. **An attitude of tenderness and softness, which brings laughter and humor into**

---

[107] www.quotery.com>quotes>quotation#226683. Dec 30, 2012.

the most difficult situations, can evoke a healing when nothing else can.

We are not born with hard hearts. I wonder when the process of hardening our hearts really begins. As we allow Life's painful situations, which we *all* face, to come into our heart and clog our arteries with plaque that hardens our physical heart, this also impacts and is impacted by our emotional heart. We humans have known about "hard hearts," and it has been written about for ages. Now we are beginning to see the *physical* results of the *emotional* hardening of our hearts, similar to the idea of open faces and closed faces. This principle is well-demonstrated by an experience that my son (David) and I shared one Sunday with our minister after church. The minister and I were talking, and ten-year-old David kept raising his hand and trying to say something. The minister stopped and said to David: "Are you trying to say something?" David then said: "I know something. Some people have open faces, and some people have closed faces. I like the ones with open faces." It is not about getting rid of the hardening of our physical heart with medications or having our arteries reamed out or undergoing plastic surgery. If we do not change our attitude, we will go right back to having a hard heart (or a closed face). *It is not about diet or exercise, it is how we face Life.* Otherwise, we will go right back to having a hard heart and/or a closed face.

For many years physicians saw patients in their living rooms, particularly in small towns and rural areas. When I practiced medicine in Wellsville, Ohio there were many times when patients were brought to my front door and examined in my living room, even though I had an office in town. Though inconvenient, it was a reality I had to deal with. I will never forget one late afternoon when the polio epidemic was rampant in Ohio. I had just returned home and taken my children upstairs for their bath and storytelling time when the phone rang. A frightened caller said that his child was very sick, and he did not know what was wrong. I told him to give me fifteen to twenty minutes to get a babysitter, and I would come by to see the child. However, in less than ten minutes, my doorbell rang and when I went to the door, he came in carrying his six-year-old daughter. He was afraid that she had polio. Since he was already in my living room, I could not send him back out, so I had to instruct my children to stay at the head of the stairs and not come down. The child did not have polio, and I was able to alleviate the father's fears and help the child.

Those of us who work as physicians are constantly faced with situations symbolized by the story I have just told. Because we have taken on this role, the living room in our dwelling place is frequently invaded by people who do not honor our boundaries. We could be in line at the grocery store, at a party or any place Life takes us. *If we are recognized in our professional role, people feel free to ask us questions and seek our advice. I know of no formula for dealing with Life on these terms.* What it requires is for us to be present and aware of the circumstances enough so that we can set whatever boundaries for ourselves that are required in the moment, like I had to do by making my children stay at the head of the stairs, so that I could then deal with the issues at hand. Life seldom separates work and personal issues in such a way that we can just "deal with things in the office" according to our plan. **Because we have chosen the profession of healing, the Universe sometimes brings to our front door issues that need to be dealt with at *that* time and place.**

I remember another time when the mayor of Wellsville came to my front door with a large laceration on his elbow. He was bleeding and in pain. I had my medical bag with me. With my children running in and out and up and down, I repaired his elbow right there on my kitchen table. Even now, though I am *officially* retired and not practicing as a physician, there is no way that I can turn my back on, or turn away from, somebody who is *genuinely* asking for help. The front door of my living room or my consciousness will always be open to people, as long as I can be of service *and* have my personal boundaries respected. My front door will also be open to new thoughts, new concepts and new experiences as long as I am consciously able to make these kinds of decisions about Life in my Living Medicine dwelling place.

Sometimes the thing that moves us out of our comfort zone is one word or phrase, such as cancer or multiple sclerosis. Sometimes it is a relationship event, such as the death of a child or spouse; or perhaps when someone moves into our home, and we must learn to readjust and accommodate them. This latter event can mean getting rid of some old furniture, moving some new furniture in or just shifting the furniture around. Sometimes the furniture that we have had for many years, which *we* think looks fine and has served *us* well, may be having problems that we do not see. For example, as a child in India, I remember times when a piece of furniture that we thought was just fine would be eaten away by termites from within. The whole piece of furniture would just crumble. We did not know what was going on *inside* of that piece of furniture, because, on the surface, it looked good. The same thing can happen with relationships in which one person feels that everything is going along well and doesn't recognize that there may be a problem. Then something happens, and the entire relationship crumbles, because it was not solid on the *inside*. This experience can also happen when a person goes into the hospital for a surgery, such as an appendectomy. Then, when their abdomen is opened up, cancer is unexpectedly found throughout. These things happen in Life, and when they do, our option is to sit back and let that particular circumstance completely destroy all the rest of the good things that have been built in this house of Living Medicine *or* we can clean up the mess, replace the furniture that has been destroyed or removed with something more useful and up-to-date.

In this war-torn world of ours, we humans can truly destroy ourselves, just as iatrogenic medicine (medicine that causes a problem by clearing up another problem) can complicate the healing process and even make it worse. The time has come when we must shift our attention from getting rid of diseases to the *true* healing aspects of nurturing and love. I believe Jesus meant it when He said: "Love your enemies" (Matthew 5:44). **If disease is one's enemy, love could make *the* difference**, as we choose *how* we deal with this guest (the disease) in our living room.

4

The Kitchen and Dining Room

In our house of Living Medicine, the kitchen and dining rooms are so open to each other that they almost resemble one unit. The reasons for this become more apparent as we look closely at this unit.

Golda Meir, president of Israel from 1969 to 1974, was a woman of deep insight with an extraordinary ability to communicate about issues in the international community in an effort to bridge gaps that remained unaddressed. She did most of her negotiations and office work in her kitchen at her dining room table. This is where she brought the heads of state from all around the world, offered them a cup of tea and some food, then began the serious negotiations. *In this family setting, while sharing food and drink, many of the hostilities that loomed so great were brought into focus in a way that allowed the perspective to shift. That way the issues could be dealt with through all lenses to reach the best solution for everyone concerned.* It is hard to hide things under a table when it is your kitchen table. There are many acceptable ways for people to hide things from one another in executive offices and corporate board rooms. This kind of communication is *very* different from the open communication that happens around a dining room table. To this day, The Foundation for Living Medicine board meetings are held around my kitchen table!

In our family, no matter what else what was going on, we all gathered together for our dinner meal every evening at six PM. During this time, we shared with each other our interests as well as our life concerns, and we all listened to each other. One evening, when my oldest son (Carl) was a freshman in college, he came home for Thanksgiving. Bill and I got started talking about the idea that the time would come when we would be able to change our genes and maybe even our basic genetic structure. The children were listening in and finally Carl, who is now a retired orthopedic surgeon, chimed in with his freshman-in-college knowledge and said: "You guys are so wrong. I have the latest scientific information about genes, and there's no way that they can *ever* be changed." He continued to expand on his latest information, when six-year-old David (who was sitting beside him and thought that the sun rose and set on the information that he got from his big brother) said: "Carl, you're wrong, and I'll prove it to you." David then jumped off his chair, ran into his bedroom and came back to stand beside Carl's chair and said: "See, I changed my jeans!" This experience taught me how important humor can be in maintaining loving communication and diffusing potential conflict. *Perhaps world peace really does start with families around kitchen tables!*

One of the central rituals in most of the major religions involves breaking bread together. Jesus' last gathering with His disciples is commemorated throughout Christendom as the Last Supper (Matthew 26:26-30). The place where our hearts open up to each other, where we share laughter and tears, where friends and enemies gather together and look at each other face-to-face can be across a dining room table. The Twenty-third Psalm, which is a major scriptural passage for Jews and Christians, also uses this ritual: "Thou preparest a table before me in the presence of mine enemies." God has prepared this table for us, a place where we can face and communicate with the enemies *outside of* ourselves, as well as a place where we can confront those aspects of our being that are our "enemies" *within*. By now, in our house of Living Medicine, we have invited people in who have become part of who and what we are. Our enemies no longer represent *only* other people or *external* aspects of ourselves. They may have also become those parts of ourselves that make us feel uncomfortable and in conflict with ourselves. These aspects are:

our fears and our hopes, which may have been dashed; our feelings about difficult people; our past pains and hurts that we carry with us all the time; or our resentments and prejudices. Our enemies can also be the things we don't like about ourselves: "My feet are too big"; "My nose is too large"; "I'm too fat"; or "I'm too thin." **Whatever it is that we see *within* ourselves that we do not like can become our enemy. These enemies can cause disease processes in our body.** Our *fears* can manifest as stomach ulcers or colitis. Our *anger* and *resentments* can raise our blood pressure. Our *jealousy* can cause heart problems, and the list goes on. In the passage from the Twenty-third Psalm quoted previously, there is *no* tablecloth being spread over the table to hide our enemies, so that we do not have to deal with them. *The fact is: at this place, at this time and in this part of our being, we are looking at and are confronted with either making friends with our "enemies" or trying to suppress them, continuing the process of maintaining our animosity towards them.*Webster's Dictionary defines "enemy" as:

1. *A person who feels hatred for or fosters harmful designs against another; an adversary or opponent*
2. *An armed foe or opposing military force*
3. *Something harmful or prejudicial*

Rather than internalizing these "enemy" aspects of ourselves, *it is critical* that we learn to deal with them in an open, conscious and thoughtful way, just as Golda Meir did. Once *we* can do this, we can support our patients (and colleagues) to face *their* "enemies" also. A few examples of this principle follow.

In his lectures and in his books, Bernie Siegel, MD[108] often shares the story of why he shaved his head following a workshop with Elisabeth Kübler-Ross in the 1970's. In that workshop, he said he had to face the truth about how miserable he was treating cancer patients as

---

[108] Siegel, Bernie S., MD. Love, Medicine and Miracles: Lessons Learned About Self-Healing From A Surgeon's Experience With Exceptional Patients, 1986 and 1998.

a successful, surgical "mechanic" ("fix this, replace that."). He shaved his head as a symbol "of the uncovering I was trying to make, baring my own emotions, spirituality and love." From that moment on, Bernie said his bald head was a constant reminder to "get involved" with his patients..."a 'cardinal sin' in medicine." He began by encouraging his patients to call him by his first name. With his wife (Bobbie) and a nurse, he started the Exceptional Cancer Patients (ECaP) program, where he dedicated *an entire day* each week to attending these groups and *just listening* to patients. By *humanizing* his medical practice, Bernie says he was able to *remain* a surgeon instead of becoming a psychiatrist! Dr. Ann shared with me that the two months of clinical training she spent with Bernie during her senior year of medical school completely changed the course of *her* life as a physician as well. "If I'd never met Bernie, I would probably have ended up becoming a plastic surgeon!" This is just one more demonstration of the power of this principle: facing our own "enemies" and dealing effectively with them not only transforms *our* lives as physicians, it can transform the lives of *others* as well.

I shared my story in the previous chapter about what happened for me when I was able to change the way I felt about my hands. Dr. Ann had a patient who had a similar "aha" moment when she attended the Body Esteem Workshop given by Rita Hovakimian in the San Francisco Bay area in the mid-1990's. Dr. Ann had referred the patient to this particular workshop because she had grown up with a mother who constantly told her she wasn't pretty/attractive because she wasn't petite and feminine, like her mother. Her mother couldn't see or appreciate that her daughter was an accomplished athlete with a strong, healthy body that others sometimes envied. Dr. Ann's patient had become so distressed by her non-petite, athletic-appearing body that she had grown to hate it. At the workshop, there was a "mirror" exercise that was clothing-optional. She told Dr. Ann that Rita had encouraged her to listen to her body and do what felt right to her during this exercise. The patient struggled with this decision, though finally decided to participate in it without her clothes. All the participants were encouraged to listen for their body's specific "message" to them. She told Dr. Ann that she had stood in front of that mirror for what seemed like hours. Finally, she "got" this message from her body: "I am *not* your enemy. I am here *only* to be in service to you." From that moment on, Dr. Ann's patient said she was *only* able to see the *unconditional love* that her body had for her, and that her previous disdain for it was *instantaneously* transformed into love and gratitude. She returned from that workshop and asked Dr. Ann to allow her to sponsor Rita to come to Seattle several times a year to give *other* women in Dr. Ann's practice the opportunity for this kind of transformative experience, which Rita did for many years thereafter. Her workshop has since become the *Women, Power & Body Esteem Coaching Certification Program*,[109] which now allows that experience to be available to women all over the world.

As we open ourselves to receiving, the kitchen/dining room area is where **nutrition and nourishment on *all* levels** of our being takes place—body, mind and spirit. The substances with which we feed these aspects of our being **create who and what we are.** For example, one of the things we have learned and know about the food we eat is that certain foods affect the "good" and "bad" cholesterol in our bloodstream. We have not really learned how much emotion and attitudes affect what we eat and how we eat, and this is something that we need to become more informed about. Cholesterol has become a big scary word, and people who know very little about their own physiology are concerned about the effects of cholesterol. The following story illustrates this point well.

A seventy-six-year-old patient was once in my office as a follow-up to a physical exam. As I gave her the results, I mentioned that her cholesterol was elevated. I did not go into a great deal of discussion about what she should do to lower it, since it was not all that high. However, she decided to take care of this problem on her own. Realizing that if she stopped eating two things that she dearly loved, bacon and

---

[109] www.inspiringsuccess.com.

peanut butter, she could probably bring her cholesterol down. Being a very wise woman, she came up with an innovative and constructive way to deal with the problem. She went with her husband and daughter to a fancy restaurant, took a candle along with her and sat down at the table. While her husband and daughter ordered their meal, she lit the candle and then ordered four strips of crisp bacon. While her family was eating, she talked to the bacon and said something like: "Bacon, I've always loved you. You've been very good to me. We've had a long and constructive relationship, but now it's time for us to part. I'm going to leave you with a great deal of love and fondness and happy memories. I'll eat two pieces and leave the remaining two on my plate, so I know that you're always here for me if I need you." After talking for a little while longer to the bacon, she blew out the candle, and they paid their bill and left. *She has not wanted bacon since that time!* I then asked her: "What did you do about the peanut butter?" She said: "Oh, that was fun. I got a new jar of peanut butter, put it on a little silver tray and walked through my home to every place I'd *ever* eaten peanut butter, singing something like this: 'Peanut butter, I love you. You've been so good to me. I have many happy memories with you, and now is the time for us to part." When she was finished, she gave the jar of peanut butter to a little girl across the street. *She has not wanted peanut butter since!* When I recently asked her about bacon and peanut butter, she said: "Oh, yeah, I haven't eaten any." The beauty of this story is two-fold: her cholesterol is now normal; *and* this wise woman was able to create a delightful ritual that allowed her, with love and caring, to let go of some foods for which she no longer had any use. She didn't say: "Oh my, I have to stop eating peanut butter and bacon. I don't know how I'm going to do it, because they're so much a part of my life." In that case, she would have created a large negative thought from out of the problem and, unable to stop, would have made them her enemies. Instead, she joyfully brought the whole problem out into the open and took care of it herself in a joyful and loving way.

As we go through life, we are continually faced with opportunities and challenges to release old habits and patterns. These habits represent emotional and physical thought patterns. They also represent spiritual mile-markers or, for those who think in these terms, "karmic trends." This can be a very painful process and one of the most difficult life journeys we will ever face, because it impacts us at *all* levels of our being. If we think that letting go of these habits and patterns is as simple as just saying "no" to them, it isn't. The attachments to these habits and patterns run too deep and usually are very long-standing. We can move forward without condemning ourselves, if we accept ourselves at our *current* level of development, recognizing that these attachments have developed *so that* we can learn and grow from them. With gratitude for what is *and* what has been, and by creating a personal ritual, we can mitigate that which needs to be released in a painless and even fun manner, as my patient did with the bacon and peanut butter. **It is only when we cling to things, whether material aspects of our lives or personal relationships, that they continue to have power over us.** The following story illuminates this principle perfectly.

I have a friend who shared a dream with me about the financial difficulties she was experiencing in her life. In this dream, she was ankle-deep in mud, struggling up a hillside to reach a swimming hole at the top. There were two small wooden carts, like the little red wagons some of us had as children. She was pushing one and pulling the other. Two of her friends accompanied her. However, *they* were skipping along and dancing and having a great time, as they all went up this hill. My friend became very frustrated with the whole process and, in a passive-aggressive way, began saying things like: "I wish somebody would help me carry this load. I wish somebody would realize how hard it is for me to push this cart, which keeps going one way or another. I wish someone would help me pull the other cart up this hill. I wish somebody would really pay attention to the hardships that I'm facing." When she looked in the carts, they were empty. She stopped in the dream and said: "Time for an attitude change." She let go of the cart she was pulling and jumped over the cart she was pushing, stretched out her arms and ran up the hill. Her friends had already let go of their loads. They were not pushing or pulling empty carts up the hill through the mud, as *they* had released theirs. Yet, she was hanging on to whatever this was that was bogging her down and making it almost impossible for her to get up to the top of the hill. She said to me: "I realize that I've been feeling like nobody's here to help me. I feel like I must carry this financial load all by myself, and I've just been having a really hard time doing this. I feel all alone. I now realize that I'm pulling an empty load. I no longer need anything that is in those empty carts. If I let them go, they will just disintegrate, and I can go on. I have no need to keep pulling this load of what probably represents self-pity, anger and resentment up the mountain. Continuing to do this is making me miserable. It feels horrible. If I let it go, I can get up the mountain and get into that swimming hole, which is where I'm headed." *We cannot really nourish ourselves until we let go of that for which we no longer have use.* We cannot add to a cup that is already full. **If we want to grow and be nourished, we first need to *let go of the old* so we can *make room for the new.***

With any attachment or addiction, when we come to a place where we must let go, we can choose the path of *karma* or the path of *grace*. If we choose the path of karma, it can become very painful and frequently has physical repercussions. If we choose the path of grace and allow the addiction to move out of our lives with God's help, we create a new pattern that leads us to a fuller and more fulfilled life. A ritual involving prayer and meditation, as well as people or friends who help us on our spiritual path, can truly relieve us of lifetimes of attachments. To move forward from there and create *new* patterns or habits that truly *support* us, Dr. Ann suggests that we consider the following principles that she learned early on in her life from Dr. Stephen Covey[110] (caps and bold are ours):

---

[110] Covey, Stephen. The 7 Habits of Highly Successful People, 1989.

KNOWLEDGE *is the theoretical paradigm, the **what to do** and **the why.** SKILL is the **how to do.** And DESIRE is the motivation, the **want to do.** In order to make something a habit in our lives, we have to have ALL THREE.*

These principles can be applied in *any* area of our life that we want to change and then create a *new* pattern or habit, just like my patient did in her dream. She could shift out of her "victim" paradigm once she *gained* the **knowledge** that both of her carts were actually empty. Then, when she realized that letting go of the empty carts was all she had to do to get to the top of the hill with ease and joy, she quickly *applied* that knowledge (*gained* the **skill**) to let go of both carts. Finally, she was able to do all this because she was *motivated* (had the **desire**) to get to the swimming hole at the top of the hill to be with her friends and have a good time.

Although *nutrition and diet* pose a perfect opportunity to deal with old habits and create new ones that serve us better in the kitchen and dining room of our Living Medicine home, that *is* not *what this book is about.* Something, however, needs to be said about the importance of basic nutrition. One fundamental tenet is that **the more we can stay with foods that are either minimally processed or not processed at all, the better our nutrition will be.** We recognize that our physical body functions better with natural or live foods, rather than those that have undergone multiple processes that kill their very Life Force. These substances include preservatives, excess sugar and salt, food colorings and any of the multitude of chemicals that alter the food from its natural state. I am certainly not suggesting that these chemically-altered foods can be *totally* eliminated from our diets. When we choose our foods, however, we can become aware of how close they are to the natural, or *living*, state in which they were produced. The whole question of genetic engineering is something that we are going to face and deal with at some time, since much of our food (worldwide) has been altered.

Some of the people I know deal with their dietary restrictions in a fanatical way. Afraid to put different types of food into their bodies, they create a state of fear. Doing this shuts down digestive juices and can actually cause more problems than partaking of that food, blessing it and being grateful for it. **It is not just the food we ingest that is important. It is also the way in which we *receive* the food, the way in which we ask our body to *deal* with this food, as well as the *total* body-mind-spirit connection we work with in digesting and absorbing the food.**

People who may or may not be concerned with the nutritional value of their food still have CHOICES which can *improve* the nutritional value of their food. One of these choices is to bless their food. **When we are grateful for what we have, our body accepts the *blessed* food with an attitude of gratitude instead of fear.** To illustrate this point, one day, when Maggie Mae (my great-granddaughter) was eighteen months old, she was with her parents, ready to eat dinner. Her mother said to her: "Maggie Mae, would you like to say grace?" Maggie Mae answered with a strong "Yes!" She closed her eyes, folded her hands and said: "God is." No more needed to be said. *That simple blessing* no doubt *transformed the food* on the table that day into something that fed not only their bodies, *it also fed their hearts and souls*, and her grandparents (who are both Presbyterian ministers) have used her statement in sermons many times since! "Out of the mouth of babes..."

Years ago, Olga Worrall, a well-known psychic and healer, did a research project in which she placed her hands around a beaker of water and said a prayer. Subsequent tests found that the water's molecular structure was changed by her prayer.[111] The progress of the scientific work with water has been brought to our awareness in

---

[111] Worrall, Olga and Ambrose. The Gift of Healing: A Personal Story of Spiritual Therapy, 1989.

great detail by Masaru Emoto, MD. His books[112,113,114] explore in-depth his theories of how water reflects at its very crystalline level the world around it—even the thoughts and words of people around it. In the movie, *What the Bleep Do We Know?*[115] Emoto shows magnificent pictures of crystals formed when water is exposed to various words and different types of music.

Since, as human beings, we are mostly made up of water, it is so important that we understand *the power of our words* in relationship to ourselves and to each other. **Kind words create beautiful crystalline structures within the water of our body, whereas *cruel* words cause disturbance and confusion, resulting in pain or illness.** When Jesus spoke of Living Water, I believe He was referring to a *physical reality* that actually manifests in response to thoughts and words of love and truth. As the Great Physician, *His* words *were able to bring healing and life to the very* molecular structure *in the bodies of the people He taught.* Knowing this helps us as physicians to understand that, **when we talk to patients, the very *words* we use bring either healing *or* more problems to them and to ourselves**. Our house of Living Medicine, both inside and outside, must be a *manifestation* of the kinds of crystalline structures Emoto's *living* water reflects. As he discovered, *water is the very essence of our being that communicates to that same essence in the body water of others.* **Thus, what gets communicated the moment anyone walks through our door is a *vibrational* message that speaks loud and clear, *with or without words*.** The actress Glenn Close understood this principle completely. In an interview with the late James Lipton (1927-2020),[116] she stated: "I love the chemistry that can be created on stage between the actors and the audience. *It's molecular* even,

---

[112] Emoto, Masaru, MD. The Hidden Messages in Water, 2004.

[113] Emoto, Masaru, MD. The True Power of Water, 2005.

[114] Emoto, Masaru, MD. The Secret Life of Water, 2005.

[115] https://whatthebleep.com

[116] Close, Glenn. Interview with James Lipton, Inside the Actors Studio, 1995. Lipton founded/hosted this program,1994-2018.

the energies that can go back and forth. I started in theater and when I first went into the movies, I felt that my energy was going to blow out the camera." The following story from my own life as an actor of sorts also speaks to the importance of this principle.

For reasons that I will explain in the next chapter, I had to repeat the first grade. During that year, our class was asked to perform a little skit before the whole student body. It included a part where "the frog jumped over the pool." Since by then I was the tallest person in the class, that part became mine. My mother made me a frog suit consisting of a shirt and pants, which she died green. I could do this part very easily, using my long legs to jump over a pan of water, which was the "pool." I walked confidently out onto the stage and looked at the audience. I immediately saw my two big brothers looking at me, which threw me off my stride.

When I jumped over the "pool," I landed right in it, much to my dismay! I stood there and started to cry when my skin turned green as my suit began to fade into the water. I was so embarrassed that I couldn't move. The teacher had to come and lead me off the stage. At dinner that night my brothers were having a great time teasing me about what happened. I was so angry at them for teasing me, though I wasn't about to let them know that. My mother listened to all of this teasing for a while. Finally she said: "All right, boys. You've had your fun. Now, *what can we do as a family to help Glady* so that, if she ever has anything like this happen again, she won't have people laughing *at* her and will have people laughing *with* her?" To this day I don't remember what we came up with. I just know that we came up with *something* which, from that day forward, has been the way I have handled embarrassing situations, which have been many! I *am* certain, though, that it was my mother's kind words that made all the difference, which the research on kindness completely supports.[117,118,119,120,121] It was recently pointed out also that, if people were approached *in a kind way* during this 2020 pandemic with the request to apply the CDC guidelines of social distancing and wearing a mask, they would be much more likely to comply with these requests than if they were approached with anger and a "guilt trip."

Similarly, it has been shown that if people *eat* while they are frightened or angry, it affects the digestive juices. One of the problems we face in this world of corporate structure is that many meetings are conducted during mealtimes, possibly causing a person to approach that meal with tension and fear, or, at the very least, in a stressed state. These emotions cause enough restriction of the digestive process that many medications (including digestive enzymes!) are sometimes prescribed to help people digest their food better and ease their symptoms. I often wonder how many of **these types of medications could be eliminated if we approached our meals *consciously*, affirming our gratitude for *whatever* food is in front of us, especially if laughter and love are also present at our table**.

It is in the kitchen and the dining room where many of the choices we make in life are manifested. **When we overeat or do not eat enough, it is a matter of CHOICE**. The food we choose, the way we choose to prepare it and the time and place where the food is served *all* affect our life and our well-being. For example, the *attitude* of the person preparing the food has a direct effect on the food. If it is prepared in anger, the food takes on the energy of anger. An example of this principle occurred with a patient I had who was so upset with the way in which her daughter-in-law did not peel potatoes "properly" that it caused a rift in her family. In this instance, my patient made a clear *choice* to use something that many of us would consider quite insignificant to create a huge upset in her whole family. Her other choice

---

[117] www.randomactsofkindness.org>the-science-of-kindness.

[118] www.kindnessevolution.org>science-of-kindness.

[119] https://ncbi.nlm.nih.gov>pmc4917056.

[120] www.honeyfoundation.org>research-and-facts-on-acts-of-kindness.

[121] www.greatergood.berkeley.edu>what-type-of-kindness-will-make-you-happiest.

could have been to accept her daughter-in-law's way of peeling potatoes as *unique to her* and let it go, to keep peace in her family and maintain a good relationship with her daughter-in-law. **In *every* moment, on issues large *and* small, our choices make a difference.**

The matter of *the relationship between Will and Choice* also needs to be addressed. To illustrate, many years ago, during one of our A.R.E. Clinic Medical Symposia, I heard Mark Thurston, PhD describe the concept of the Will, and I have never forgotten it. He likened our movement in consciousness to a sailing vessel, with the rudder of the ship representing the Will. The rudder keeps the ship on track and allows it to get to its destination (life purpose or ideal). Constructed of strong enough material, it is not easily bent or destroyed by heavy seas or the storms of Life. The rudder is controlled by the person guiding the ship, and that person is manifesting choice. *Every choice made by the person in control of the rudder either brings the ship closer to its destination or takes it farther away from it.*

The difference between **Choice** (which is manifested in the second spiritual center or the cells of Leydig) and the **Will** (which is manifested in the fifth spiritual center or thyroid) is a matter of structure and function. **Our ability to choose directs the way our Will allows us to follow our chosen path.** If our goal is to achieve Oneness, both within ourselves *and* to return to our original state of Oneness with the Creator, then it is only through the *conscious* use of Choice in directing our Will that we can accomplish that goal. Our Will must be strong enough to respond to the choices that we make. Thus, accomplishing our goal hinges on the cooperation between our individual choices and the way those choices direct our Will. **It is only as we create *cooperative* action between our physical, mental and spiritual bodies that we truly manifest a *balance* in our lives, and it is this balance that allows us to be *whole*.** We cannot truly manifest God's Will in *this* world without having the physical aspect of *our* Will functioning harmoniously and in balance *with Choice*. This principle can best be illustrated with the following story about one of my patients who is now also a very dear friend.

Eveline is in her mid-seventies and has suffered with severe pain for many years. She is very sensitive to prescription medications, thus, pain medicine is *not* her choice for controlling her pain. Her nature is that of an artist, and she lives her life that way, seeing and creating beauty in *everything*. A few years back, she realized that she needed to find some way of dealing with pain that would allow her to live her life more fully, so she came up with what she calls *"pain*-ting." To Eveline, this term means that when the pain gets so severe that she feels it is almost intolerable, she finds *something* to paint. This "something" could be her shoes, her purse, her wall. It could also be a piece of material that she has just found which she will then make into a dress, a blouse or some other useful object. Even a simple piece of paper can be transformed into a *pain*-ting. She gets out her paints and paintbrush and then starts painting, *losing herself in what she is creating, until the pain becomes tolerable again*. She calls this "putting the *ting* back into [her] painting." Through the years of living with her chronic pain condition, Eveline has created the most beautiful home for herself. Her backyard has a long stone wall along its border, and she has created a beautiful scene on each portion of that wall. Over time, her *pain*-tings have evolved into a truly lovely mural, which now spans the entire wall. When you meet this lovely lady, you would never know that she suffers with chronic pain.

Cooperation involves much more than just working with our body. It also involves the everyday choices of partnering with other individuals and cooperating with the energy of the earth and the entire Universe. This principle was never made clearer to me than when I was at a conference in Council Grove, Kansas in 2006 where Mietek Wirkus and his wife (Margaret) presented a workshop describing the research they did at the National Institutes of Health.[122] As a healer and energy worker, Mietek had conducted a study while he was in Poland and had been continuing it since he came to the United States. His work included energy research for the purpose of healing people. He had been asked by the National Institutes of Health to research

---

[122] www.mietekwirkus.com

cells and cellular structure. The NIH was particularly interested in the way individual cells absorb their nutrients, specifically in relationship to how they absorb calcium, *after* the cells had been exposed to Mietek's healing energy. What the studies demonstrated was that the cells which were exposed to Mietek's healing energy absorbed twenty-two percent more calcium than prior to their exposure to his energy. The fact that Mietek demonstrated he could increase the uptake of calcium in cells with the use of healing thoughts and healing intention is important. He did this consistently and repeatedly.

Since we now know it is possible to use energy in this way, we now also know that *we* can increase the calcium absorbed by our *own* bone cells. *With our intention and our thoughts, we can make stronger bones!* Telling women to fight osteoporosis as though they are going to fight their own bones may be causing more pathology in their skeletal structures than we realize. Understanding that **thoughts are things**, and that **the cells in our bodies really *do* know what to do *and* how to do it**, is truly **what Living Medicine is all about.** This principle became very real to me one day when I went to see Susan Kramer, a patient with whom I had also become friends, at a hospital rehab center. Susan had been in an automobile accident two months prior and had so severely injured her spine that she was lying in a full body cast with her head and neck immobilized. She was unable to move any part of her body except her eyes and mouth, so that healing could take place. All she could do was lie flat and look at the ceiling. At first, Susan was fed through tubes, though soon was able to ingest liquids and semi-solid foods through a straw. She had friends bring soups and healthy foods to her in the hospital. When she was told that her chances of recovering to the point of even being able to sit up were remote, she prepared herself for a life of almost total disability. I explained to her the role that the osteoblasts and osteoclasts play in bone regeneration—that one of the cells was created to remove debris, while the other was designed to rebuild bone tissue. Here is how she describes what happened next (bold is mine):

*Dr. Gladys McGarey came to visit. She told me to talk to my cells—that they would know what to do. I couldn't remember exactly what she said when she visited me, but I do know that [she said] I had to talk to myself. **I told my cells to fix what needed to be fixed.** I think, when my body was repairing itself, I must have been on automatic pilot. The fractures at the lower part of my spine were healing while I was lying flat on my back for four months, immobile.*[123]

Susan was finally able to move her head a little. She began to sit up and, when they were able to perform X-rays, her physicians found that *her spinal column was beginning to heal.* She was able to go home after four months and, six months after that, she said: "I'm home. I can walk. I even opened a jar. My fingers are working better. I walk in the pool every day. The last X-ray showed that my neck is healing. I even now have a normal curve in the curvy part of my neck, which was flat. The doctor feels I'll soon be [able to wear] a soft collar, and [may] even be able to turn my head." As of the publication of the second edition of this book, Susan has been able to return to the weekly meetings of my study group, driving herself to and from them. Although Susan is not yet *completely* pain-free, she now lives her life fully and joyfully. *With her attitude, her mind and her nutrition, Susan was able to repair damage that the medical community told her was impossible to repair.*

I had dinner with Susan a few months later. She had driven her own car to the restaurant and sat upright in her chair. The day before our dinner together, she had done a rigorous, round-trip, one-mile hike with a friend into Montezuma's Well (an underwater well fed by an aquifer that is a former limestone sinkhole). To our dinner, she wore a soft collar support decorated with a beautiful necklace. She removed the collar during dinner, demonstrating that she could hold her head up straight, without support, for short periods of time. She told me that after she got home from the hospital, a friend of hers had

---

[123] From personal correspondence to Dr. Gladys.

performed some energy work and craniosacral adjustments on her. These treatments eased the discomfort that had been so severe in her scalp that even the slightest movement of air caused her sharp pain. *The devastation Susan's body had suffered was as severe for her as Hurricane Katrina had been to New Orleans.* When I talked to her further about her stay in the hospital and the time when she was unable to do anything *except* visualize mental pictures, she told me the following remarkable story.

Susan said that when she moved her eyes to the *right,* she saw New Orleans being completely rebuilt. She kept focusing on this city that had been so horribly devastated and recreated it in her mind, street by street and house by house. She even saw the color of the houses and the way the city was being rebuilt. **Using visualization, her body** began to understand that it, too, **could rebuild.** She saw the rebuilding of New Orleans as symbolic of the rebuilding of *her* body, cell by cell and structure by structure. Susan then said, as she moved her eyes to the *left,* that she saw an ancient city with a stream running through it and buildings that lined its banks. She saw the color of the buildings, as well as their structure and stability. She did not know where this city was, yet she knew it existed. About three months later, when Susan was home and watching the Discovery Channel, she said she saw a picture of Bern, Switzerland, and recognized it as the city she had seen in her visualizations! In Susan's mind, this picture of the city of Bern was a symbol of the underlying pattern of her healing. She recognized the stability and beauty of this city and incorporated those images into the rebuilding of her body. At the time, I was not aware—nor was she, I'm sure—of the *NLP research on eye movements.*[124] This research demonstrates that looking to the *right* is a "constructed imagery" (future-focused) process, and looking to the *left* is a "remembered imagery" (past-focused or memory) process!

Virginia Veach, PhD was a psycho-oncologist, psychotherapist and educator who traveled the world delivering comfort and healing to thousands of people in difficult circumstances. During the Vietnam

---

[124] www.nlpu.com/Articles/artic14/Eye Movements and NLP by Robert Dilts, 1998.

War, she went to a camp with a group of fourteen other people where they brought hope and healing to severely neglected people who had very little to eat and nothing in the way of support. After her team spent time with them and shared what they could, the village people wanted to do something to let Virginia and her group know how much they appreciated their help, so they prepared a meal for them. The village people each put one grain of rice in the common bowl. In this manner, they collected enough to create a sparse meal. Since water also remained very scarce, the villagers had one bucketful in which they washed their hands and the dishes, serving that *same* water to all the people in her group to drink. Since this meal and water were offered to them with love, they put aside any fears about bacterial contamination or illness that might result from drinking such contaminated water. As a result, *not one* of her group experienced *any* symptoms or any illness from drinking the village's water or eating their food.[125] When I heard her tell that story, I could not help but glory in the wonderful reality that was manifested through love and gratitude. This story also demonstrates **the power of *belief***, as this group *truly* believed that *the love present was* stronger *than any harmful bacteria* that might have been in the food and water they consumed. Bruce Lipton, PhD[126] has done groundbreaking research in cell biology and quantum physics to show that **our bodies *can* be changed as we retrain our thinking**.

Some people live by themselves and do not have family or friends to share the dining experience with. For them, it would be ideal to create an environment of health and happiness as they fix *their own* meals and eat them. However, it is important to emphasize that *how* people do this is a very individual choice and can look quite different from person to person. Preparing food for oneself and eating *consciously* in this way is an opportunity to show love and gratitude *for*

---

[125] www.Commonweal.org>tns>podcasts

[126] Lipton, Bruce H., PhD. The Biology of Belief: Unleashing the Power of Consciousness, Matter and Miracles, 2005 and 2015.

ourselves, as Gabriel Cousens, MD discusses thoroughly in his book *Conscious Eating.*[127]

The *physical* kitchen, with all its appliances—be they chrome-plated fixtures, *just* an electric stove, a modern refrigerator with an ice maker or an open fire over which food is cooked— is *not* what is vital to the way in which food is prepared and presented. Although I have a fully-functioning electric kitchen at this point in my life, I remember as a child having the food prepared over an open fire with no running water available. Instead, our water had to be boiled and stored in containers for drinking. Some of the best meals I ever had were prepared in that manner. Since there was no refrigeration in the jungles where we lived, the food had to be consumed immediately. **In Life, we need to learn to adapt and work with whatever condition we are faced with as it arises**. If we don't, we might become angry and frustrated. Should this happen and negative thoughts creep in, *our food may* not *be contaminated with bacteria, although it* can *become contaminated by an* attitude. **Food that is prepared by an *angry* person carries with it the vibration of *that* emotion and *cannot be as healthy* as food prepared by someone with a loving, joyful attitude.** I have friends who are so obsessed with keeping bacterial contamination out of their food that they use *chemicals* almost constantly to keep all surfaces they come in contact with bacteria-free. In the process of doing this, I wonder how much the food is contaminated by the chemicals that are used to kill the bacteria itself! I wonder whether *the attitude of people who are so intent on destroying life forms (such as bacteria) may be preserving food that is unhealthy for* them *and* also *for the people who eat the food* they *prepare.*

The food that goes into our bodies should be clean, yet not sterile. Our kitchens should *also* be clean, and they do not need to be sterile, either. The conditions in the outdoor kitchen where I grew up were certainly *not* sterile, yet, *we were healthy!* I remember times as a child in the jungles of India when we would come across *dakh* (roofed bungalows that served as outposts for the British soldiers).

---

[127] Published in 1992, updated in 2000.

These buildings sat in a remote part of the jungle where the officers were stationed and rarely saw other people for months on end. It was part of their discipline, as well as part of just maintaining their sanity and sense of direction, to maintain their customs. For example, they dressed for dinner *every* night. They ate at *exactly* the same time, exercising great care about their manners. When *we* lived in the jungles of India, though, we were much freer and more relaxed about our dining etiquette. We weren't allowed to be careless and sloppy. There were times, however, when laughter and storytelling would *completely* take over proper table manners, and we would be caught up in the life of the situation. When we would return to town, we would have to try and tame our wild spirits, and my mother would say to us: "Now just remember, you're not in the jungle anymore."

In our house of Living Medicine, we need to be aware of what our life is *really* about. We need to identify what is *important* in our life and what will increase the Life Force within us. In so doing, the life we live becomes an abundant one, as we learn to adapt to each and every circumstance. **How we choose to eat *physically*, feed our *minds* and nurture our *spirits* is truly what keeps us *alive*.**

As my children were growing up, we would always gather around the dining room table. There were many times, since my husband and I were both physicians, when our dinner conversations would deal with some specific medical problem or issue. Perhaps that is one of the reasons all six of my children chose healing professions! The food that they ate was "contaminated" by thoughts and ideas associated with the field of medicine. That was not a *bad* thing, it was just the way life was in *our* household. The children brought their lives to the table, including their friends, and we brought ours. *As we all shared our day-to-day life experiences* together, *we understood each other better.* One thing I insisted on though, no matter what else was going on during the day, was that at six o'clock at night, we gathered around the dining room table for dinner. Many were the times when I was called away during a meal because a baby was about to be born. Bill was also sometimes called away because a patient needed care.

Many were the times when something was said at the table that hurt someone's feelings and that person may have left the table because they were upset. However, the times that we *really* remember are those where we laughed so hard we could hardly sit up, or when the puns that were created were a challenge for us all.

As physicians, we need to take our patients' histories, including asking them what their diet is like, which is very important and frequently overlooked. In so doing, we can help them understand the importance of *sharing their life experiences* in an open and healthy way, both with us as well as with those closest to them. I know of no better place or healthier situation for them to learn to open up about their life experiences than when sharing a meal with others. As we dine with our table companions, bringing *our* memories together with each of *theirs* in an open and caring way, *each one of us* has the opportunity to experience healing in whatever way we *individually* need. As a daily practice, this experience can bring life and health to all who gather in this way to break bread together and share from their hearts. As the *patient's* Physician Without and as *our own* Physician Within, we are in a unique position to encourage this kind of healthy ritual to the Physician Within each patient, as we *both* **recognize and acknowledge the importance of shared experiences**.

5

The Library

In my home, my library sits adjacent to my dining room. It is so full of books that they are stacked on all the shelves and on the floor. It seems to me that these books keep reproducing themselves! I give books away and more books appear. Many of the books are precious to me because of being personally autographed. Others are precious because I have read them many times, and they have a special message and meaning for me. Still others are precious because they are old—they are treasures because of their antiquity. Some even belonged to my parents.

There are also many books in my library that I have *not* read, yet they are still precious to me, because they are in my life, and I know they are there. These books are about philosophy, music, humor, hope, fear, excitement and passion. So many of the emotions and experiences that we humans have are depicted and written about in these books. You might say that *my library is my own personal history*. It is so updated that I even have my computer in it! In addition, my parents' medical diplomas are also hanging on the walls, along with a picture of Elisabeth Kübler-Ross, MD with Mother Teresa. My awards, my diplomas and my family pictures also hang on these walls.

Although small, there is so much history packed into this room that it really serves as *the central part of my home* of Living Medicine. The futon pulls out to create a guest bed, so life is not just about what has happened in the *past* in my library, it is also about what is going on *right now* in my home. *It is my present, my future and a record of my past.* It is also where we buried the time capsule when I built this house. In addition, this is the place where I do my writing. It is where I can call up old memories, like some of my old books that may not have been visited for years, and create new ones. "Just as breathing exercises help integrate body and mind, writing is a kind of psycho-neural muscular activity which helps bridge and integrate the conscious and subconscious minds..." states Stephen Covey.[128] As we have collaborated together to write this second edition in this safe, sacred space in my home, Dr. Ann and I have both *consistently experienced* what this prolific author has also observed: "writing distills, crystallizes and clarifies thought and helps break the whole into parts." The following two stories illustrate well, I think, why I choose to do my writing in this room.

Writing, in general, has always been very difficult for me. There are at least two reasons for this, I think: the first is because I am an author, *not* a writer, and the second is because I am dyslexic. I became aware of the difference between authors and writers some years back. **Authors** have a message that they *need* to write about, yet often find that task quite frustrating and difficult to accomplish. **Writers**, on the other hand, feel a deep *compulsion* to write—they *must* write—much like the feeling of needing to breathe to live. My dyslexia no doubt contributes to my being an author instead of a writer. Its impact on my life is quite another matter, however, and I think my story is worth sharing here in detail.

My symptoms of what was diagnosed much later in my life as dyslexia became readily apparent to me between the ages of six to nine years old (1926-29), when I was a student at the Woodstock School in the Himalaya Mountains. *During this time, there was no diagnosis of a condition called dyslexia, though that condition was as much a part of my life as my name.* I had difficulty reading words, as well as adding and subtracting numbers. I was considered the class "dummy" in first grade. In fact, I had to repeat that grade, because the word *god*

---

[128] Covey, Stephen. The 7 Habits of Highly Successful People, 1989.

and *dog* looked **exactly** the same to me. Because of this then name-less affliction, school became an experience of *daily torture* for me. My *only* relief from it resided one thousand feet up the mountain in the form of my Ayah. Each day after school, she was there waiting for me, following my steep, uphill climb home. Sitting on her haunches, wrapped in her rough, woolen, drab-green shaw, she would hold out her arms to me and, in Hindustani, say, "Come here." She would wrap her arms around me, and I would be covered by her shawl. She knew I was a sad little girl—and I was—as well as an angry one. *Under Ayah's shawl, though, I knew I had a place of safety and healing.* There, in that sacred space under her shawl and in the safety of her arms, I stayed for as long as I needed. That simple gesture and those precious moments with her gave me what I needed to face another day in school. I have kept that homespun shawl for more than ninety years now. My *current* place of healing and safety is in the protected, sacred space of my library, where I also recuperate and prepare my-self to meet my next life struggle, which is why I do my writing there, dyslexia and all!

India was torn apart in 1947. The conflict between the Hindus and Muslims had erupted. My parents and my physician brother (Carl) were in India then, doing what they could with the tools available to them. They were inoculating against disease, patching up wounds, setting bones, treating malaria, helping with the birthing of babies, handing out cures or remedies for other maladies, and even digging graves for those who had lost their lives in India's struggle. Mahatma Gandhi was also there, giving his breath, energy and life to help his people come to an understanding with each other. He was working for the healing of his beloved country with the tools *he* had, in much the same way that my parents and brother worked with *their* healing tools. A friendship and a great deal of respect developed between my parents and the Mahatma. He gave my mother a shawl made of blue Kashmiri (cashmere) wool. It was much different from the one that my Ayah wore. However, this shawl given to my mother came to repre-sent yet another safe place for me: the sacred space that Mahatma

Gandhi held in his heart for his people. When I am in my library, surrounded by *my own* writings as well as those of my holistic medicine colleagues, it is the sacred space where I hold in my heart **the vision of Living Medicine: transforming "killing" medicine into a *healing* paradigm for *all* humanity.**

What these two shawls carry with them and have in common are love, caring and compassion. One represents the love of a simple, illiterate woman for a troubled little girl. The other reflects the love of a great man for millions of people in his troubled country. They are *both* treasured possessions to me to this day. On very special occasions, I wear the blue one; taking with me the *healing energy* of those who made it, those who wore it and the reason why it was given to my mother. When I wear the shawl my Ayah gave me, the feelings of *safety* envelop me, no matter what life struggle I may be dealing with in the current moment. When children cling to their tattered blankies, they know this feeling of finding a safe place in the presence of these simple objects that carry great power through the love they represent. Viewed in this way, *taking blankies away from children* before *they are ready to give them up would be a sacrilege*!

Having been born and raised in India in the foothills of the Himalayas, I always wanted to see Mt. Everest and never really had the opportunity. So, in 1990, when my brother (Carl Taylor, MD) invited me to accompany a group of physicians doing some work with the village people in Tibet, I was thrilled. The Chinese and Tibetan governments had asked him to bring a team back into the villages to identify the health problems of the local inhabitants. We went to a village that was at fourteen thousand feet elevation and a little farther away from Mt. Everest than we had hoped. Still, Everest should have been in plain sight. However, since it was July and also the rainy season, clouds covered the mountains the whole time we were there. As we prepared to leave, I thought: "Well, I will just have to come back another time, because I'm not going to get to see Everest this time." Then, as we were driving back on the bus, for some reason, *a voice inside me said*: "Turn around." I did so, and for a short period of time, the clouds separated, and there it was! I yelled "There's Everest!" and the bus driver slammed on the brakes. By the time we got out to take a better look, though, the clouds had closed, hiding it from view. Nevertheless, we had seen Mt. Everest! For me, it was like a transcendental experience, because no one can ever tell me that I have *not* seen Mt. Everest! In my heart, I know Mt. Everest is there, and I know that I had that experience of seeing it, and it was unusually deep and meaningful.

When I got back home, I wondered why seeing Mt. Everest was so important to me. Then I happened to pick up the book that my father had written (see preface). In it was one small chapter, just one page long, which began with the statement: "When our trio was to become a quartet..."— which meant that my parents already had three children and I, the fourth, was on the way. Dad goes on to say that he and Mom took a trip by horseback to Simla in the Himalayas. During that trip, they wanted to get a glimpse of Mt. Everest. Because of the clouds, however, they were unable to see it. I then realized what my experience of seeing Mt. Everest was all about: even in utero I was trying to get a glimpse of Mt. Everest and had not been able to, and now I had finally seen it! **We store memories from this lifetime and past lifetimes in our consciousness so that, when needed, they can be accessed and made available to us.** My father's book with the one-page story about Mt. Everest brought the experience of my intra-uterine life into perspective with my trip in 1990. This glimpse of Mt. Everest will now always be a part of my *conscious* personal history as well as my *unconscious* intra-uterine experience.

One of the exciting treasure hunts in my library has been to find evidence of *my own* evolving timeline in the field of medicine. Bill and I started our medical practice in Wellsville, Ohio in 1948 and practiced there together until he was called into the Air Force as a flight surgeon during the Korean War in 1951. I practiced alone in Wellsville until June 1955, then I moved to Phoenix. Bill had already been in practice there with Jack McCarville, MD at the Wagon Wheel Shopping Center on 40th Street and Thomas Road. for five months and continued to practice with him there until January of 1958. During this interim, I was pregnant with my youngest daughter and struggling to get my Arizona medical license. It was being held up because I was born in India and had no *original* birth certificate. It took a letter from Paul Singer, MD (President of the Maricopa County Medical Association) to the Arizona medical board, instructing them to quit harassing me. He told them to give me my license, because doctors—*especially women physicians*—were in short supply in Maricopa County. They grudgingly issued it. Bill and I were then able to join our practices once again, requiring us to move up to 56th Street and Indian School Road in Phoenix. That was the *only* year I was not actively involved in a *full* medical practice until I retired in 2004!

In 1957, Bill met Milton Erickson, MD at a medical meeting and became very much interested in Milton's work with hypnosis. So, we decided to invite a few medical colleagues to meet with Milton who shared our interest in learning more about alternative ways of practicing medicine. Since Milton was well known in the field of hypnosis, we decided to start working with his concepts. To get started, we invited three other MD colleagues to our home on a Tuesday night in the summer of 1957: Robert Watterson, James Berens and Bill Rogers. Our little group continued to meet every Tuesday night to learn from Milton about how we could use his techniques in our medical practices. The sessions would go on well into the night because the topic was so exciting and relevant to what we were learning. During this time, I was pregnant with our daughter (Helene) and still struggling to get my Arizona medical license. By the middle of August when I was eight months pregnant, these late-night meetings were becoming hard for me, so I asked that they move the meeting to another location. In doing so, they came up with a name for the group: **The American Society of Clinical Hypnosis**, which still exists by this name today.

Francis Sarikowski, MD joined our practice in 1963, and the three of us built the building for the Olive Tree Medical Group. In 1964, we moved our practice to 40th Street and Indian School Road in Phoenix. Her life partner, Eleanore Schafer, CAC joined us at that time and worked with patients who had addictions.

In 1969, Bill and I joined Hugh Lynn Cayce (Edgar Cayce's eldest son) on the first around-the-world trip with the Association for Research and Enlightenment (A.R.E.), the organization formed in 1931 to study and research the work of Edgar Cayce. There were about forty people with us on this trip. One night, after we had spent the day at a kibbutz outside of Jerusalem, Bill and I spent the night talking about *evolving the Olive Tree Medical Group into the A.R.E. Clinic.* There were four A.R.E. board members from Virginia Beach in the travel group, including Hugh Lynn Cayce. We presented them with the concept of changing the way we had been practicing medicine into a research-oriented A.R.E. clinic. When the members of the board returned to Virginia Beach, they presented this idea to the entire board, who unanimously approved our proposal, and *our practice became* the *A.R.E. Clinic.*

In the early 1960's, Bill and I decided to spend some time alone one weekend in Apache Junction, Arizona. We had been working very hard and needed the time to rest. When we awakened one morning, Bill had had a dream that was so vivid that we both felt we had to follow up on it. He dreamt he was coming down a staircase and, at the end of the staircase, Hugh Lynn Cayce was waiting for him with a message. He said to Bill: "You need to start an **Academy of Parapsychology and Medicine.**" As we sat down to breakfast, we began to think of how we could create this type of academy. We decided that we needed some person other than one of us to be its president. We had just heard a stirring lecture given by Robert Bradley, MD about his new book[129] and thought Bob would be the perfect person to do this. So, we wrote him a letter and told him what we were thinking. We received an answer back that was six pages long! The first three pages outlined all the reasons why he could *not* do it. In the middle of the third page, however, he said: "Well, why not?" He then became

---

[129] Bradley, Robert A., MD. Husband-Coached Childbirth: The Bradley Method of Natural Childbirth, published in 1965, 1979 and 2008.

president, Richard Miles became secretary, Robert Mattson became treasurer, and now we were off and running! *All through the 1960's and 1970's, the Academy of Parapsychology and Medicine presented* monthly *workshops up and down the West Coast.* We dealt with all the emerging ideas about health and healing. There would sometimes be a thousand people in the audience at a time when the whole world was alive with anticipation and hope, as a new paradigm shift in consciousness began to emerge.

Prior to this dream, Bill had been writing a monthly newsletter entitled *Pathways to Health* (no longer in print). Physicians who were interested in these emerging ideas would subscribe and write to us about things that were going on within their lives and practices. Laypeople could also subscribe and receive this newsletter. One day, sometime in 1967, we received a letter from a mailman in Maine. He said that he had received our newsletter and was very interested in his own health and healing. He mentioned he had been in an accident three months prior and had injured his ankle very badly. No one could find out what was wrong with his ankle. He was off work because he could not walk his route and was looking for healing. In the *Pathways* newsletter he had read that if you have a sore throat, it helps to put a castor oil pack around your neck (to open up the lymphatics), which will frequently help to clear a sore throat. He said he had *had* a sore throat, so he had put the castor oil pack on his *neck*. Much to his surprise, his *ankle* symptoms cleared up, and he now had complete return of function in his ankle! He wanted to know what had happened. Bill and I looked at each other and said: "We don't have a clue!"

In the next newsletter that went out, Bill wrote about this man's story and said: "If there's anybody out there who knows what happened here, please let me know." We got an answer from a doctor in Italy (Ian Urquhart, MD) who said: "If you guys knew anything about *acupuncture*, you would know that the bladder meridian starts in the head, goes down the neck to the ankle and onto the toe. When the energy block was removed in the mailman's neck by the application of the castor oil pack, it cleared the bladder meridian, which removed the energy block in the ankle and brought about the healing in the ankle." Bill and I looked at each other and said: "What is this acupuncture?" We then embarked on the journey to learn about this ancient form of healing.

President Nixon had just gone to China and seen some amazing surgical procedures done there using acupuncture as the *only* form of anesthesia, so it seemed that the world might be ready to hear more about it. We wrote to Felix Mann, MD in Great Britain, who had written five books on acupuncture. We wrote to people in Germany and Italy, as well as people in Taiwan and Japan. Our search led us to learn enough about acupuncture that we were able to teach the basic principles during the workshops and lectures presented at the Academy of Parapsychology and Medicine. These workshops led to our creating the *very first* **Symposium on Acupuncture** *in the United States*, which was held at Stanford University on June 17, 1972. Two hundred eighty-five practicing physicians were in attendance! **We taught what we knew**, and the physicians who picked up that knowledge used it and grew with it, and *now acupuncture is an accepted therapeutic modality in most healing centers in the United States.*

In 1977 a group of us physicians felt that we needed to form an association to give voice to the aspects of medicine we were all talking about, writing about and working with. There were five of us who decided to meet in Hemet, California to talk in-depth about creating this organization. Evarts Loomis, MD had a center there called Meadowlark, and he hosted us for a five-day conference. Besides Evarts and me, the other attendees were: Norm Shealy, MD; Gerald Looney, MD; and Bill McGarey, MD. We decided to call our organization **The American Holistic Medical Association**. We elected temporary officers at that time with Norm Shealy as president, me as vice president and Gerald Looney as secretary-treasurer. We also chose a date (1978) and place (Denver, Colorado) for our *first* national conference, so that we could present ourselves *officially* as a medical association. We decided that the officers would maintain their positions for two years. It took us those *entire* two years to decide how to spell "holistic" (with an "h" or with a "w"?)! It was only after we realized that the word we were looking for came from the root word for *health, holy and healing,* that we finally agreed to spell holistic with an "h"! Yearly medical meetings have been held ever since, which have brought together physicians from all over the world who are furthering the vision of holistic medicine. The AHMA then morphed into the AIHMA (the American *Integrative* Holistic Medical Association). Many members thought this was a more inclusive title, while others considered it redundant...much like the "w" vs. "h" discussion! The organization *still* exists to this day, though it morphed again into the AIHM (the Academy of Integrative Health and Medicine), which now allows *all* holistic practitioners to have membership and be recognized. *It is no longer a physician-only organization.* The jury is still out on whether this was the *best* next morphogenesis of the organization or not, especially from a physician's point of view. Personally, I can see both sides of this perspective, and only time will tell if *this* morphogenesis moved the needle forward or backward to "legitimize" holistic physicians.

Dr. Francis Sarikowski left our A.R.E. Clinic to start her own practice in 1972. Bill and I continued to work together at the A.R.E. Clinic during the remainder of the 1970's and 1980's. Many physicians of all ages joined us along the way. We continued the journey of discovering and practicing holistic medicine, including the Cayce concepts, along with the *best* of the conventional medicine of the day. In addition to incorporating acupuncture into our entire practice (including birthing), we created the "Baby Buggy" program, which allowed for safe and loving home births and taught parents how to have healthy families. We also taught many ten- and fourteen-day live-in programs. *Creative Living* was the ten-day one, which I organized and led; *Temple Beautiful* was the fourteen-day one, organized and led by Bill. These in-house programs showed people how meditation and other self-help methods could assist them to discover their *individual* life purpose (ideal). They were also designed to help them create a lifestyle to support them in their life journey, which may or may not have included some specific illness or disease process. In addition, we held the *annual* A.R.E. Clinic Symposium to explore and work with what were considered "complementary" medicine concepts at that time. In conjunction with our conventional and holistic approaches, we also incorporated nutrition, biofeedback, massage, dream therapy and stress-reducing/centering activities (including yoga, *tai chi* and breath work), *as well as* the Cayce remedies[130] (including the many uses of castor oil and castor oil packs)[131,132] *and* advanced osteopathic principles and practices (including Sutherland's cranial-sacral techniques).

As I was going through some old papers, I came across an editorial printed in the *Journal of the American Medical Association* on September 5, 1986 quoting one of its prior editorials from September 4, 1886 (the year my osteopathic physician father was born!) entitled "The Higher Education of Women." It states:

> *A good professional education is very expensive...not alone...of money, but...of physiological force; much more than a woman can afford, if she is to perform her proper functions as a producer of men...The production of children calls for far more physiological force on the part of the mother...The functions of gestation and maternity require a great outlay of physiological force, and if this force is used up in other work, the offspring of the world must suffer, as must the woman herself.*
>
> *While it may be true that too much bodily labor may render a person less prolific, it is very*

---

[130] McGarey, William A. MD. The Edgar Cayce Remedies, 1983.

[131] Baar, Bruce, MS, ND (editor). Castor Oil Pack Therapy: Application and Instruction, 2016 (4th edition).

[132] Heritage Store. The Palma Christi Castor Oil Pack Kit (cold-pressed, hexane-free), www.amazon.com.

much more clearly shown that excessive mental labor is a cause of sterility... In its full sense, the reproductive power means the power to bear a well-developed infant, and to supply that infant with the natural food for the natural period. Most of the flat-chested girls who survive their high-pressure education are unable to do this... Our education, our civilization, is one that stunts, deforms and enfeebles women... Shall we make it worse by placing women in competition with men, by still further stunting, deforming and enfeebling her animal powers?

This article, published in THE medical journal of the day, may seem laughable to us now; however, these were the deeply-held convictions of *most* people at that time, *not* just physicians. The exciting aspect of this awareness comes into focus, though, when we look at the way medicine was practiced over a hundred years ago and how we have progressed since then. Women are no longer considered "baby machines," although many happily accept the role of motherhood as *part* of their lives. In addition, nearly half (47.9 percent) of the students who graduated in 2019 from medical schools were women![133] It should also be noted, to Andrew Taylor Still's credit (the founder of the American School of Osteopathy in 1892), *nearly one-third* of the *first* class of osteopathic medical students (who were granted DO—Doctor of Osteopathy—degrees instead of MD degrees) were women![134] Nearly one hundred and thirty years later, more than half (51.2 percent) of all *osteopathic* medical *applicants* are now women[135] (actual *matriculated* female medical student numbers for 2020 are still in the

---

[133] www.aamc.org>2019-facts-enrollment-graduates-and-MD-PhD-data(2019).
[134] Quinn, Thomas A. The Feminine Touch: Woman in Osteopathic Medicine, 2011.
[135] www.AACOMAS.org>applicants-by-COM-and-gender-2019-2020.

process of being calculated). And, as of 2019, half (50.5 percent) of all matriculated MD students were women.[136]

The following is a part of my personal history that many people may not know: because *both* of my parents were osteopathic physicians (DO's), I would have been one also if the Reformed Presbyterian Church had allowed DO's to become medical missionaries to ndia in 1941. My reason for going to medical school was to follow in my parents' footsteps. To do that, I had to become an MD! The only reason my parents even got to be medical missionaries as DO's was because my father took what we would today consider to be a residency in eye surgery in Los Angeles. He graduated from that program with an MD degree, and thus likely became the *first* DO/MD in this country...all because he wanted to be allowed to go to India as a medical missionary! My DO mother would not have been allowed to go with him as a medical missionary had she not been married to him! Talk about fate! However, this was the *end* result of their *individual* fates, as their following personal stories will explain.

My father (John Calvin Taylor, Sr.) was a Kansas farmer and the eldest of five children. His father was injured during the Spanish-American war (1898). In 1910, when his younger brother was old enough to take over the running of the farm, my dad applied to medical school in Chicago. He had always dreamed of becoming a physician, and now he had the opportunity to get the education that would allow him to do so. When he swung his suitcase up into the train on his way to Chicago, he twisted his back and was walking down the aisle with a limp. An elderly man watched as he came down the aisle and called out to him, asking him why he was limping. When my dad told him what had happened, this gentleman said to him: "You know, we're going right through Kirksville (Missouri) on this train, and there's a physician there who's started a new medical school. He calls his work osteopathy, and he's done some amazing things to help people with problems like yours. I'd suggest that you stop off and have him

---

[136] https://www.aamc.org/news-insights/press-releases/majority-us-medical-students-are-women-new-data-show.

look at you and see what he can do." My dad took this kind man's suggestion, got off the train in Kirksville and went to see Andrew Taylor Still, DO. Dr. Still treated my dad, and his recovery was so remarkable that my dad stayed on in Kirksville, entered *osteopathic* medical school and got his DO degree in 1912!

My mother, Elizabeth Siehl, had lived all her life in Cincinnati, Ohio. Like my dad, her dream was also to become a physician. She worked as a seamstress to help support her family. One day, she was sitting on the front porch of the family home and observed her neighbor walking down the street *without a limp*. My mother was very surprised to see this, because she had always known this lady to walk *with* a limp. She went running to greet her neighbor to find out what had happened. Her neighbor was very excited to tell my mother her story. She said that there was a new doctor in town who called himself an osteopath. He said he had gone to school in Kirksville, Missouri and learned this type of healing from Dr. Andrew Taylor Still. My mother immediately got as much information as she could from her neighbor, wrote to the school and was accepted. Her dream was about to come true, as she boarded the train and went to Kirksville. She became an osteopath in 1913.

My parents met in medical school, were married in 1913 and went to India as Presbyterian medical missionaries in 1914. They spent the rest of their lives bringing healing to the village people of North India. They started a children's home for the children of leper parents, and there are thousands of healthy people in *all* parts of the world now who grew up in this children's home. My dad's younger sister (Lorena Belle Taylor) also became an osteopath and worked with my parents in India. She died in the Bhogpur area of North India and is buried there. My mother's younger brother (Walter Siehl) was a prominent osteopath all his life, working in Cincinnati, Ohio. Five of his six sons became osteopaths. Donald Siehl was his oldest son and the *first* osteopathic orthopedic surgeon in this country. *I have often wondered if that elderly man on the train was an angel of some kind.* It was he who set my father on the path that he was clearly destined to fulfill. My dear mother would not have been able to fulfill *her* destiny had my father not chosen to follow that call to osteopathy in Kirksville in the early 1900's and met my mother there. Bless that man, whoever he was, for giving me such a rich heritage from which to draw and make *my* contribution and mark on the world of medicine! Thank goodness that I have lived long enough to see my profession begin to bring *feminine* energy back into the practice of medicine!

Ancient traditional medicine has always known that *true* healing must be accompanied by nurturing, support and encouragement. I believe this goal is best accomplished with *feminine* energy in the picture. When medicine assumed the role of fighting diseases that attack from the outside, it became something that required *masculine* energy to create the instruments through which we destroy disease. **If all our energy is directed towards *destruction*, however, we will never win this battle against disease. *Feminine* energy allows us to rebuild, reconstruct and reactivate the *spiritual* essence of who we are.** It becomes apparent that we need to emphasize and re-awaken the gentle, compassionate, healing energy that is manifested in the *true* feminine, which is called Love.

Focusing on the relationship of body, mind and spirit is *one* of the main messages of Living Medicine. The role that women play in reawakening the value of this principle is something we *now* recognize. ***True* healing needs to embrace a *balance* of our male and female aspects.** Without the presence of the feminine face of medicine, we would continue to just *fight disease* and not have the participation of the *spirit* as part of the healing process. This balance is **what is needed to raise our two-dimensional bodies into third-dimensional consciousness.**

I have heard it said (paraphrased): "Women are taught to shrink to fit."[137] It is encouraging that we can now laugh at the concepts held a hundred years ago and see that we really *have* made progress in the way we approach the healing of the body, mind and spirit. This

---

[137] www.goodreads>author>11291>Chimamanda>Ngozi>Adichie

principle was brought personally home to me years ago when my sister visited me. We went with my daughter (Helene) to the cemetery where my mother and father are buried. When Helene saw the memorial plate on their grave, she was incensed and said: "Mom, how could you do that?" I did not know what she was talking about until I looked again and realized what I had put on the memorial plate: "Dr. John C. Taylor" and "Elizabeth S. Taylor." No "Doctor," no DO title and no acknowledgement of the fact that my mother was a doctor, too! I have since corrected that mistake, and the plate now reads: "Elizabeth S. Taylor – Pioneering Doctor and Mother to the Children." In that moment, we both realized *how much* things had changed through three generations!

When Mother and Dad were introduced in a group, it would go something like: "This is Dr. John Taylor and his wife, Elizabeth, who is also a doctor." When I was introduced with my husband, both of us being physicians, the person making the introductions would ask me: "Do you want to be introduced as Dr. Gladys McGarey or Mrs. Bill McGarey?" I would say: "It doesn't make any difference. Both are all right." The issue was not important to me at that time. However, in the *third* generation when my daughter (Helene) was introduced with her husband (also a doctor), she would *never* be referred to as Mrs. Fred Wechsler—she was *Doctor* Helene Wechsler, and there was no question about it! So, *within three generations, the shift from women physicians being thought of as a "tagalong" or, worse, being* completely *unacknowledged as a physician, to now being* recognized *as a physician in* her own *right is very apparent and totally accepted.*

As we see the re-emergence of the feminine in the field of medicine, we also become aware of the path that conventional medicine has taken. When I was president of the American Holistic Medical Association in 1982, I received a letter from one of our trustees (Walt Stoll, MD) in which he gently reprimanded me for using the term "nontraditional" regarding our work. He suggested that we accept our position as the *true* traditionalists in medicine, and that the current practice of medicine should be termed "conventional." Walt's position was that the kind of medicine that is taught today should be called *conventional* medicine, since it deals primarily with the scientific diagnosis and treatment of diseases. The holistic physician of today is *really* the "traditional" doctor. Why? Because we are working with, and trying to understand, the *total* human being and how his or her lifestyle, thoughts and beliefs affect or create their illness or health. We, as holistic physicians, work with concepts and methodologies that are steeped in tradition. We, in the field of holistic medicine, are doing the things that have always been accepted as the role of the "traditional" physician. Acupuncture and herbal medicine are certainly traditional. Manipulation and massage have been known and used since the beginning of time. Castor oil was used for Cleopatra by her physician. Prayer, meditation and the laying-on-of-hands have been practiced by physicians for thousands of years. The power of healing associated with the "song" of the Native American shaman has been important in that culture, along with many other healing techniques, for eons. Their definition of medicine is life. The research that documents this historical information has been wonderfully summarized in Dan Benor's *Healing Research* series, Vols 1,2,3.[138]

As "traditional" physicians, we may use alternative healing techniques; however, we do not *just* practice alternative medicine, so we would technically be considered *complementary* medicine physicians. There are those aspects of medicine shared by *both* the traditional and conventional disciplines, such as surgery and obstetrics. As we update the concepts of traditional medicine, we bring to conventional medicine the dimensions of the Spirit and creative thinking, plus the *modalities* that are traditional in nature and often called "alternative." It has only been during the last two hundred and ten years that traditional medicine has been moved from the center of the medical stage and allopathic concepts of conventional medicine have taken its place. It was in 1910 that the Flexner Report was created and implemented,

---

[138] Benor, Daniel (MD, PhD). Healing Research – Vols 1,2,3 – Spiritual Healing: Scientific Validation of a Healing Revolution (2000), Consciousness, Bioenergy and Healing: Self-healing and Energy Medicine for the 21st Century (2004), Personal Spirituality: Science, Spirit and the Eternal Soul (2006).

bringing medical education from the apprenticeship model into the universities which, in turn, moved allopathic medicine into its present scientific, clinical format. Certainly, Imhotep, Hippocrates, Osler and the biblical Luke all wrote about concepts that were clearly holistic. Maimonides, a Hebrew physician who lived from 1135 to 1204 AD, said: **"The physician should not treat the disease, but the patient who is suffering from it."**[139] In modern times, one of the great medical writers, Félix Martí-Ibáñez, MD (1911-1972), had this to say: "To be a doctor, then, means much more than to dispense pills or to patch up or repair torn flesh and shattered minds. To be a doctor is to be an intermediary between man and God."[140] *As holistic physicians let us not forget to claim our heritage as the real traditional physicians and RE-claim the feminine face of medicine.*

These historical distinctions and experiences are all part of *my* personal and professional evolving timeline and history. **What Living Medicine does is to bring the *Life Force* back into the established practice of medicine.** Holistic medicine merged body, mind and spirit. **Living Medicine** infuses *Life itself* into the practice of *all* forms of medicine. It **brings traditional medicine *back to life* and asks conventional medicine to become a *living* thing**, because *to be well-trained is* not *the same as being well-educated.*[141] To be well-educated means taking the training we have received and putting it into action within *our own* lives. To use training *without* education can be dangerous, as we have witnessed repeatedly in the allopathic model with its focus on *killing* medicine instead of *living* medicine.

I consider **the foundation of Living Medicine** to be **the five L's: Life, Love, Laughter, Labor and Listening**. What activates *all* of them, though, is the *Divine* Spark, which is the *unconditional* Love with which God created the world and *all* living things. As *consciously-evolving* human beings, we are constantly striving to allow this Divine Love to manifest *through* us *to* all living things.

---

[139] Rosner, Fred. The Medical Legacy of Moses Maimonides,1998.

[140] Félix Martí-Ibáñez, MD. To Be a Doctor, 1968.

[141] https://keydifferences.com>difference>between>training>and>education

- **Life**: If we are not alive, nothing else matters. Without *love*, life cannot exist. *With* love, the Spark of Life is activated.
- **Love**: Love is the energetic force that runs through *all* of the L's. It is akin to the "dominant" thread in a hem, which holds *all* the other stitches together and which, if pulled, will cause the *entire* hem to unravel. Without the "dominant thread" of love, there is no *true* healing; and *with* it, the healing process is activated. That is why we may cure a disease and *not* heal the patient **or** heal the patient without curing the disease.
- **Laughter**: Laughter sits right in the middle of the five L's. Laughter *without* love is cruel. *With* love, it brings the energy of joy and hope into our lives. It makes our lives juicier and helps us with the next step.
- **Labor**: Without labor, the first three L's cannot manifest on this dimension; and labor, by itself, is just too hard and dry. Without *love*, labor becomes drudgery. *With* love, it becomes bliss, which gives it purpose.
- **Listening**: It is important to listen to ourselves, our own body, the world around us and to each other. Listening allows the healing process to move outside of ourselves to the world around us *and* bring the outside world into our own healing. Without *love*, listening is empty sound. *With* love, you can actually *hear* the message and not just the sound.

I was talking to somebody about these concepts a while back, and they said: "Okay, so what about gratitude? What about hope? What about forgiveness?" I said: "They are the *outcome* of the 'fruits of the Spirit.' They are *some* of the building blocks we use to build the *structure* of Living Medicine upon the foundation of the five L's." To illustrate: The American writer, Augusten Burroughs[142] said: "If you have your health, you have everything.

---

[142] www.augusten.com.

When you do not have your health, nothing else matters at all."[143] I have heard this quote repeated many times and spoken as one of the truths that people accept. *I think that Living Medicine goes beyond this statement.* I have many patients who have physical issues, emotional issues and even spiritual issues that they work with. Yet, because they have life and claim life, they have everything. I would like to change that statement to say: "If you have *life*, you have everything," because **being healthy is the process of *living* life and adjusting to *all* its gifts, including the ones that are smooth and easy as well as the difficult ones.** Unfortunately, *we are often so busy trying to prevent death that we are really* killing *life*.

Light is the Spark that activates Life, which must be nurtured by Love. The rigid "i" in Life represents the *masculine* aspect of the Life Force or the "I AM that I AM" kind of strength that is stable and immovable. It needs to become aware enough to allow itself to soften, bend and move into the round "o" in Love. Love now represents the *feminine* or more nurturing aspect of the Life Force that can become a wheel, allowing Life to then go on and on. Otherwise, **Life without Love would wither and die,** as science has now well-demonstrated in a significant longitudinal research project (the Grant and Glueck studies[144]). In this project, "the physical and emotional well-being of two populations [was tracked for over seventy-five years]: 456 poor men growing up in Boston from 1939-2014 (the Grant study) and 248 male graduates from Harvard's classes of 1939-1944 (the Glueck study)."[145] The significance of the findings in these studies is so relevant to the tenets of Living Medicine that we decided it was important to report them in detail here (bold and caps added by me for emphasis).

---

[143] Burroughs, Augusten. Dry, 2003.

[144] www.adultdevelopmentstudies.org.

[145] Curtin, Melanie. "This 75-Year Harvard Study Found the 1 Secret to Leading a Fulfilling Life" (see www.inc.com).

Due to the length of the research period, [multiple generations of researchers were] *required. Since before WW II, they diligently analyzed blood samples, conducted brain scans (once they became available) and pored over self-reported surveys,* [in addition to annual personal] *interactions with these men, to compile* [their] *findings. Their conclusion? Ac-cording to Robert Waldinger, director of the Harvard Study of Adult Development, one* [outcome surpassed] *all the rest in terms of importance—the clearest message that we* [got] *from this 75-year study is this:* **good relation-ships keep us happier and healthier. Period.** *NOT how much is in your 401(k). NOT how many conferences you spoke at or key-noted. NOT how many blog posts you wrote or how many followers you had or how many tech companies you worked for or how much power you wielded there or how much you vested at each. No,* **the biggest predictor of happiness and fulfillment overall in life is...love.** [The study specifically found the **key components of love** to be **someone to rely on** and **the quality of one's close re-lationships**]*...how much* VULNER-ABILITY *and* DEPTH *exists within them; how* SAFE *you feel sharing with one another; the extent to which you* CAN RELAX *and* BE SEEN *for who you truly are and* TRULY SEE ANOTH-ER. [In addition, the data also showed that] ***those who feel lonely are more likely to see their physical health decline earlier and die younger.***

[In the words of] *George Vaillant, the Harvard psychiatrist who directed the study from 1972-2004, the two fundamental elements to explain* [these findings] *are as follows: "One is love. The other is finding a way of coping with life that does not push love away."This is a very good reminder to* **prioritize not only connection but your own capacity to process emotions and stress.** *If you're struggling, get a good therapist. Join a support group. Invest in a workshop. Get a grief counselor.* **Take personal growth seriously** *so you are available for connection. Because the data is clear that, in the end, you* [can] *have all the money you've ever wanted, a successful career and be in good physical health, but* **without loving relationships, you won't be happy.** [So] *the next time you are scrolling through Facebook instead of being present with your significant other, or you're considering staying late at the office instead of getting together with your close friend, or you catch yourself working on a Saturday instead of going to the farmer's market with your sister,* **consider making a different choice.** *"Relationships are messy, and they're complicated" acknowledges Waldinger. But he's adamant in his research-backed assessment: "the good life is built with good relationships."*

Thus, we can now answer, with utmost certainty, the question posed in that famous Tina Turner song: "What's love got to do with it?" As it turns out...everything!

At this age in my life, I am just beginning to understand something about the way my mother and father loved me. My father's love was more like a bright, sunny day. For him, understanding *and* speaking the truth were both very, very important. My mother's love, on the other hand, was more like a refreshing spring breeze with the scent of orange blossoms. I experienced these differences one day while we were sitting in my garden, just two weeks before my mother made her transition. My mother said to my father: "John, look at that petunia plant. It must have four hundred blossoms!" My dad said: "Oh, Beth, there can't be more than forty." My mom's response to him was: "What's another zero?" I knew that they were both telling *their* truths

from *their own* perspectives, even when my mother added the per-
fume of orange blossoms to her truth. They *both* loved that petunia
plant in their own way, and they *both* experienced it differently.

So it is with living and loving. **As individuals, we are constantly changing. As long as we are alive, we have the opportunity
to grow.** Each one of us experiences growth in our own particular
way and has the opportunity to share that growth with those we love.
Some thoughts expressed by Cassandra Clare in one of the books in
her series *The Shadowhunter Chronicles*[146] captures this concept well
for me (italics are mine): "There is truth in stories. Fiction is truth, even
if it is not fact. If you believe *only* in facts and forget the stories, your
brain will live, but your heart will die." Last, though certainly far from
least, Alice Roosevelt Longworth (1884-1980) sums it up the best, I
think: "I have a simple philosophy. **Fill what's empty. Empty what's
full. Scratch where it itches.**"[147] If that isn't **the best Rx for Life,** I
don't know what is!

A great portion of my library houses books containing the information derived from the Edgar Cayce readings. In fact, huge areas of
space would open up on my shelves if I were to remove the material
that has its roots in his work. Edgar Cayce was a humble man who
was born in 1877 in rural Kentucky and died in 1945 in Virginia Beach,
Virginia. He is, perhaps, the most well-known (and, certainly, *the most
well-documented*) psychic of our time. Cayce had the astonishing
ability to move into an altered state of consciousness and contact the
unconscious mind of the person for whom he was giving a "reading."
More than fourteen thousand of these readings have been studied in
detail and are housed at the A.R.E. in Virginia Beach, Virginia. For
most of his lifetime, Cayce received requests for help for all kinds
of problems —physical, mental, emotional and spiritual—from people
who would write to him. Then, from this state of altered consciousness, he gave them readings to explain why the condition existed

---

[146] www.cassandraclare.com

[147] https://quotes.thefamouspeople.com>25>memorable>quotes>by>alice>roosevelt
>longworth (Theodore Roosevelt's daughter).

and what they could do about it. Some nine thousand of the readings were termed "physical," which meant they dealt with health problems. These readings included aspects of disease and therapeutic modalities that were sometimes unusual, as well as those considered very conventional at that time.

The depth and breadth of Edgar Cayce's work has provided an ongoing source of information and inspiration for me. For example, way back in the 1930's, he talked about *individual* cells having consciousness. So, when I understood that **every cell of our body is a conscious entity,** I was then able to see that the body is really a *community* that works with the mind and spirit in the healing process, and that *all* healing begins at the cellular level! The Edgar Cayce material also brought the concept of reincarnation into focus for me. When the idea of reincarnation became part of my thinking, I already had four children. Two more (Helene and David) came into our home after I had learned something about how to prepare for pregnancy, with the concept of reincarnation giving me a broader view of life.

Helene and David are two years apart. Both talked about possible past lives as easily as they discussed their lives in school. However, it seemed that emotions always played their part as well. As David's older sister, Helene picked on him from the time they were both little, though they became the best of friends in their teens. Those early years, though, were sometimes stressful. One day, when Helene was about eight and David was six, they had one of their usual spats. Most of the time, Bill and I let them settle these things by themselves. This time, however, their spat seemed to be getting a little more heated between them, so I took David aside to talk to him while Bill talked to Helene. Bill said to her: "Now, Helene, you know you chose this family and, sooner or later, you're going to have to learn to get along with David, or you'll come back as his wife or something." Quick as a flash, she responded: "Yes, I know that, but that's before I knew David was coming!"

When Bill and I first became interested in the Edgar Cayce material, it was very difficult for us to understand Cayce's approach to diseases. Due to our training in medicine, we looked for a diagnosis of specific diseases and the therapies that would help us to treat them. *Edgar Cayce's approach to healing did not fit this model.* It was only after repeated, gentle pushing from Cayce's son (Hugh Lynn Cayce) that we began to understand that this approach was *not* focused on the disease; it was focused instead on the *person* and the physiological principles inherent in maintaining health. Cayce talked about a *balance* between the kidneys and the liver, *coordination* between the sympathetic and the parasympathetic nervous systems, as well as the importance and proper functioning of the lymphatic system. When we finally understood Cayce's approach to diagnosis and treatment, we were able to comprehend that the use of the castor oil pack for problems as *divergent* as epilepsy and a sprained ankle had a great deal to do with the *optimal* functioning of the lymphatic system. Edgar Cayce's readings identified a person's specific disease(s), though the treatments he prescribed for them were *very* individual.

I have been asked repeatedly if I treat multiple sclerosis or breast cancer, or some other disease. My answer to that question is: "No. I do, however, treat *people* who happen to be struggling with multiple sclerosis or breast cancer or hepatitis, or whatever their issue might be." It is also interesting to note that the *only* diseases mentioned in the Bible, as far as I know, are leprosy and epilepsy. *Jesus did not treat diseases, He healed people.* When the woman with the bloody flow touched the hem of His garment, there was no mention of fibroids or menopause or cancer or any other disease entity. It was simply the *symptom.* The Bible does not describe the man with the withered arm who was healed on the Sabbath as having polio or brachial plexus syndrome or any other disease process. Again, it was simply the *symptom.* Jesus, of course, as the Great Physician, was able to **see beyond the *symptom*** to the issues which that particular soul was dealing with. The healing came about when He said: "Your sins are forgiven you. Go and sin no more."

Forgiveness can certainly be one of the possible energetic forces to break the bonds holding the blocked patterns in place that can cause illness. The Chinese say that pain comes from blocks in the *chi* energy, and acupuncture allows this energy to flow again, relieving the pain. Castor oil packs clear the lymphatics, so that the lymph can flow once again without obstruction. Cayce recommended the wet cell and impedance devices as early as the beginning of the twentieth century. These instruments were effective in balancing and moving energy within the body to initiate healing in the various parts of the body. *The field of energy medicine has expanded exponentially since.* We know, psychologically, if we allow ourselves to be blocked emotionally, it becomes very difficult for us to proceed with life. **Fear and anger block energy. Laughter, music and beauty shift that block and allow the energy to move again**.

When we view these concepts in the context of the Life energy that rises along the path of the kundalini through the seven spiritual centers, then we begin to see that if the energy becomes stuck at the level of the adrenals where judgment, lack of forgiveness, anger and, particularly, fear reside, *true* healing will not manifest until the energy moves through the adrenals and rises up into the heart chakra. This is the spiritual center where love, compassion and forgiveness dwell. The Bible says: "God is love" (John 4:8), and Jesus came to earth to manifest the love of God in the flesh. It is when we, as individuals, can manifest the *consciousness* of the Christ that *true* healing can come to *us* and to the earth. Sometimes this means that, as in the case of the Apostle Paul, there may still be a "thorn in the flesh" or some symptom that may not be eliminated…yet, we can *all* still experience healing. My mother's way of dealing with such "thorns" was to be nonjudgmental: "There is so much good in the worst of us, and so much bad in the best of us, that it hardly behooves *any* of us to talk about the rest of us."[148] In conventional medicine, we have many tools to evaluate even the most unusual of symptoms. However, **if we ap-**

---

[148] Hoch, Edward Wallis (1849-1925). The Marion (Kansas) Record, owned by the author and assumed to have been written by him, per Jennie E. Taylor's article "Did Edgar Cayce Really Say That?" (www.edgarcayce.org>A.R.E.>AboutUS>Blog, December 14, 2018).

proach patients *without* compassion and *true* caring, they may never have a chance to experience the possibility of *true* healing.

My library is probably the place where I learned more about *patience* and *consistency* than in any other room. I am not very much into the Computer Age, and the use of the computer (including Zoom in this time of being quarantined at home during the 2020 pandemic!) has been a *process* in which I have often lost patience and have had trouble remaining consistent. However, the computer is *still* in my library, because I am *persistent* in my efforts to learn how to use it better. **The importance of living life in the present—day by day, line upon line and precept upon precept—allows for the possibility of *true* healing to occur.** It *must* happen at a cellular level. It *must* happen as an *ongoing* process. These three words: *patience, persistence* and *consistency* are PIVOTAL to understanding and working with the Cayce material *and* life. For years, I have heard people complain that this material is very difficult to understand, with its long sentences and archaic language. Yet, I know that if we put patience, persistence and consistency into action, we will be able to understand on a deeper level what Edgar Cayce had to say. Simply looking at and reading the words can be very confusing and does not begin to touch the *wisdom* available to us from this material. **We must look deeper than the "fix-it" consciousness to bring about *true* healing.**

We all have times in our lives when patience becomes necessary. I experienced this during the time when my oldest daughter (Analea) started writing my biography. She completed the manuscript, and we felt that the work was done. To our amazement, much of the work had quite literally just begun! *Patience, persistence and consistency were all necessary to get the work done up to that point.* We were then faced with releasing our control over the work. We had to turn it over to the publisher, editor, printer, cover designer and bookbinder, with little or no control over the time involved to create the final product. If we thought it was going to take two months, it usually took four. If we were told that certain parts of the process had been completed, we assumed that things would go faster; they did not. Finally, when we were told it had gone to the bookbinder and would probably take a couple of weeks to complete, it took three months. Now, in retrospect, the end product was well worth it, and our *impatience* with the process was only a waste of energy and totally unfruitful. However, if any of the steps along the way had been eliminated to fit our expectations, we would have had an *incomplete* product and, in reality, it would have been like having a *premature* baby.

Jesus said: "In patience, possess ye your souls" (Luke 21:19). *Impatience probably causes more strain and stress in our lives than any one thing.* We get impatient with ourselves, with our loved ones, with Life itself and with situations that do not go the way we think they should at that particular time. Our blood pressure rises, our anger builds, our adrenals get exhausted, and I even think we *age* faster! If I had a lesson to learn about patience while publishing that book, my lesson about patience seemed much more challenging when the book was dealing with healing. *We are impatient people by our very natures.* We want to grow up too fast until we are older, and then we become impatient with the aging process and want to be younger! *True* **healing requires LEARNING TO ADAPT TO CHANGES—***physically,* at the cellular and molecular levels; *mentally,* by changing our attitudes and thoughts; *emotionally,* by working with our feelings to bring them to resolution; **and** *spiritually,* by attuning to the Divine. If we try to bypass or speed up the process at *any* level, it is like interfering with a pregnancy and not allowing the baby to grow at *its* own rate, to meet *its* own needs, so it can be born as a *full-term* baby.

There is a story about a man who found a butterfly's cocoon. One day, a small opening appeared in the cocoon. He sat and watched the butterfly for several hours, as it struggled to force its body through that little hole. Then, it seemed to stop making any progress. It appeared as if it had gotten as far as it could and could move no further. So, the man decided to help the butterfly. He took a pair of scissors and snipped off the remaining bit of the cocoon. The butterfly then emerged easily. However, it had a swollen body and small, shriveled wings. The man continued to watch the butterfly, because he expected that, at any moment, the wings would enlarge and expand to support the body that would contract in time. *Neither of those things happened!* In fact, the butterfly spent the rest of its life crawling around with a swollen body and shriveled wings, *never* able to fly. What the man, in his haste and attempted kindness, did not understand was that the restricting cocoon and the struggle required for the butterfly to get through the tiny opening was God's way of forcing fluid from the butterfly's body into its wings so that it would be *ready* for flight once it achieved its freedom from the cocoon.

Sometimes struggles are *exactly* what we need in our lives. *If God allowed us to go through our lives without any obstacles, it would cripple us.* We would not be as strong as we *could* be. We would *never* fly! If we can begin to understand that Life is a *process*, that everything we do is *part* of that process and that we learn *only* as we accept the ongoing reality of that process, we can then begin to relax and enjoy life. **This is the very essence of Living Medicine.** Patience and joy go hand in hand. *It is hard to be impatient when you are laughing!*

We are so accustomed to *immediate* success for healing that it remains very difficult for us to have *patience* with a healing that may take a long time. **For *true* healing to happen, we must allow *sufficient* time and patience, while working with the *process* of healing.** *Practicing persistence and consistency can bring* any *issue into focus.* This is our *conscious* job, then we must have *patience* to complete it. It is like planting a seed and then watering it. We do this *consciously* and consistently, then we must *patiently* let it grow. If we keep digging it up to see how it is coming along, we kill it. In Cayce's words, patience is "the impelling influence."[149]

In our experience, the principle of *persistence* is often misunderstood. We hear it used in conjunction with the word "try," a word that is mostly thought of in a *negative* way in the context of persistence. For example, we sometimes hear people say: "Trying" to pick up a pencil doesn't result in the *actual* picking up of the pencil; it's only used as

---

[149] www.edgarcayce.org. Readings 262-25 — 262-27.

an excuse *not* to pick up the pencil. "Stop 'trying'—just DO it!" is the most common phrase used in this context. However, in the way that Cayce used the word "try," I think of that word as an important part of the principle of *persistence*. Using the above analogy, if I want to actually pick up the pencil, I must *first* have the INTENTION to pick up the pencil ("mind is the builder" per Cayce). Then I need to start taking the *steps* to pick up the pencil. This is where the *act* of "trying" comes in: if *actually* picking up the pencil is viewed as reaching the *top* of a ladder ("the physical is the result" per Cayce), then "trying" is taking the steps I need to take *to get to* the top of the ladder...*the steps needed for me to be able to* pick up the pencil! Our culture diminishes "trying" instead of recognizing it as *part of the journey*. Where the principle of *persistence* comes in for me in this analogy is this: we must KEEP ON *putting one foot in front of the other* AND climb *every* step of the ladder, or we won't make it to the top to pick up the pencil! **As physicians, we need to give our patients *and* ourselves credit for "trying" *any and all* steps that it takes to bring about *true* healing.**

Our library holds our memories, which can be accessed as we look for answers and search for therapeutic modalities for *both* ourselves and our patients. In 1982, I was asked to speak as president of the American Holistic Medical Association at a conference for clinical psychologists in Washington, D.C. These folks represented the leaders and "teachers of the teachers" in this area, and ten thousand psychologists were expected for this international gathering. The president of the American Medical Association and I were scheduled to speak for thirty minutes each, and then the session would open for questions. I wrote to the AMA president, Dr. Rial, twice on our gold-embossed AHMA stationery, suggesting we speak to each other beforehand to get a better sense of each of our talks. *He never answered my letters.* I was concerned by this, because the AMA was considered such an important organization, while the AHMA was just a fledgling one. The idea of facing that many psychologists in my position of being *in opposition to* the president of the AMA was really intimidating to me. I asked my study group to keep me in their prayers constantly.

That same weekend, I was also speaking at an A.R.E. meeting in Washington, D.C. At the end of my A.R.E. talk, I asked the attendees to pray for me when I spoke to the psychologists. Then, I left the A.R.E. meeting and went to the hotel where the psychologists were gathered. It was a Sunday afternoon, and Dr. Rial and I were scheduled to speak Monday morning. Sunday evening I decided to go down to the opening meeting of the organization, so I would get a sense of what was expected and a feeling for the group itself before I spoke to them. I sat in the back row of that huge auditorium, feeling overwhelmed by *both* the size of the audience *and* my responsibility to adequately convey the message of the AHMA the next day, wondering what in the world I was to say. Finally, feeling smaller and smaller, I felt that if I did not go back up to my room, I would just fall through the floor. I really asked for God's help to say and do the best I could. I went back up to my room and could not sleep, so I picked up the Gideon Bible and turned randomly to Proverbs 11:14, which says: "Where no counsel is, the people fall; but in the presence of a multitude of counselors, there is safety." After reading this statement, I said: "Thank you, God" and slept like a baby!

The next morning, I had breakfast with Jean Ann Caywood, who was the executive director of the AHMA at that time. I was still feeling very insecure about giving my presentation within the next hour. Just as we were finishing breakfast, a woman approached us and said: "Something terrible has happened. While Dr. Rial was flying from Baltimore to Washington D.C., his plane was caught up in a windstorm, and his plane had to turn back to Baltimore. He couldn't land. *He won't be at the meeting.*" This news was *a great relief to me*, as I now had an entire hour by myself to do my presentation about holistic medicine! In closing, I told the group about Proverbs 11:14 and said: "And you, my friends, are a multitude of counselors." With that, they were on their feet with a standing ovation!

Group and individual prayers are surely answered one way or another, we just do not understand *how*. Sometimes our prayers are answered with a "yes" and, at other times, God simply lets us know that the answer is "no." Or God may answer in a form that we have *not* expected and maybe do not appreciate. Also, *God's timing and our timing are not always the same.* With Dr. Rial, I would never have expected the prayers to be answered in that way. I have heard of snowstorms, hailstorms and sandstorms delaying flights; however, I have *never* heard of a windstorm during a short-distance flight (such as from Baltimore to Washington, D.C.) that was so strong that the plane had to turn back! *I believe it is impossible to overestimate the power of prayer.*

Much like the memories gathered and placed on the shelves of our physical libraries, habits *are the memories stored in our bodies, as our bodies are the libraries for our thoughts and emotions. The following story* is a great example of this principle.

Years ago, when my sister (Margaret) was visiting me, we became aware of a mannerism that we both shared. Something would happen and, without saying a word, we would each take one hand and just sweep it to the side in exactly the same way. We started to wonder why we did this, because there did not seem to be any reason for it. We realized that we both usually made this gesture at a time when we were responding to something that had taken place. We said to each other: "Why do we do this?" We had no answer. So, we pondered this question together: "Who do we know that used to do this?" We both recalled that it was our mother. Our next question was: "Why did she do this?" We realized she did it when something happened that she chose not to give much energy or attention to. She would take her hand and just sweep it to the side, essentially meaning: "Don't pay any attention to this" or "It doesn't make any difference." What we learned through our mother's action and her words was a way of dealing with issues that could be irritating and confusing. We could just let them go, accept that they were there, then release them with this movement of our hand. I know that I was able to deal with difficult situations in my life throughout the years by simply making this one gesture, even though I was not *consciously* aware of it. When something happened that was uncomfortable, uncalled for or just unpleasant, I realized I could *choose* how to deal with it. Instead of taking it into my heart and saying: "Oh my, that's terrible...that's very bad, I don't like it," I could merely let it go by making this gesture. Then I could just go on with what was important in my life at the time. I could also choose to *focus* on the issue and *not* let it go. Rather than choosing to focus on what could be a real dilemma, my mother taught us to accept the reality that *sometimes problems* do *happen, and it is just better to let go and move on.*

The Chinese do something very similar during their *tai chi* practice. They take the energy that comes *towards* them and, instead of confronting it and making it a major problem, they just accept it. To do this, they take the negative energy that is coming towards them into the palm of their hand, then let it drop off as they move their hand to their side. In so doing, they let the negative energy simply pass by them, moving it out of their lives. Since that time, I have talked to many of my patients about these techniques and have found that using them has helped them deal effectively with life's irritations, instead of letting these irritations confuse them or cause them conflict and become major problems in their lives.

Another mannerism that I have become aware of is the way I use my hands in times of conflict. If I have something that I disagree with and lift my hands with my palms pointing *away* from my body as I say "no," it becomes an act of defiance or confrontation. However, if I lift my hands and have my palms facing *towards* me, this motion can be translated into something like: "I don't think so" or "That's not right." This latter gesture allows my opinion to be expressed without engaging in an act of confrontation. It does not feel the same to me when my palm is facing *towards* me as it does when my palm is facing towards the person to whom I am speaking. It also has been said that the eye of God is in the palm of our hand. So, when I use this technique of turning my palm *towards myself,* instead of having it face the person with whom I am disagreeing, I reclaim *my own energy* by having it come back to me *without* confronting the other person. It allows me to have a conversation that is ongoing and healing with another person, instead of a combative or destructive one.

The following story shared on Facebook was reportedly told by Rehan Allahwala,[150] a Pakistani business magnate and the founder of Super Technologies, Inc and the Institute of Peace. It was reportedly presented in a motivational talk he gave in Karachi, Pakistan on January 19, 2014. This story demonstrates yet another very powerful way of dealing with potential problems or conflicts in our lives: **the value of *reframing* one's perspective, then acting accordingly** (bold is mine).

One day a farmer's donkey fell down into a well. The animal cried piteously for hours as the farmer tried to figure out what to do. Finally, he decided the animal was old, and the well needed to be covered up anyway; it just wasn't worth it to retrieve the donkey. He invited all his neighbors to come over and help him. They all grabbed a shovel and began to shovel dirt into the well. At first, when the donkey realized what was happening, he cried horribly. Then, to everyone's amazement, he quieted down. A few shovel-loads later, the farmer finally looked down the well. He was astonished at what he saw. With each shovelful of dirt that hit his back, the donkey was doing something amazing. He would shake it off and take a step up. As the farmer's neighbors continued to shovel dirt on top of the animal, he would shake it off and take a step up. Pretty soon, everyone was amazed as the donkey stepped up over the edge of the well and happily trotted off!

---

[150] www.RehanAllahwala.com

MORAL TO THIS STORY:

*Life is going to shovel dirt on you, all kinds
of dirt. The trick to getting out of the well is to
shake it off and take a step up. **Each of our
troubles is a steppingstone. We can get
out of the deepest wells just by** not stop-
**ping AND never giving up! Shake it off and
take a step up!***

Remember the five simple rules to be happy:

1. *Free you heart from hatred—forgive.*
2. *Free your mind from worries—most never happen.*
3. *Live simply and appreciate what you have.*
4. *Give more.*
5. *Expect less from people and more from yourself.*

*Sometimes it is faith and trust that is required of us in times of
dealing with Life's challenges.* When I feel misunderstood, discouraged, or impatient to achieve a goal I have set for myself, I pull out the
following story from my library shelf. It reminds me of who's *ultimately*
in charge of the "big picture" of my life, which is often a view I cannot
see in those moments.

Just P.U.S.H.

*A man was sleeping at night in his cabin when
suddenly his room was filled with light, and
God appeared. The Lord told the man He had
work for him to do and showed him a large rock
in front of his cabin. The Lord explained that
the man was to push against the rock with all
his might. So, this the man did, day after day.*

For many years, the man toiled from sun up to sundown, his shoulders set squarely against the cold, massive surface of the unmoving rock, pushing with all his might. Each night the man returned to his cabin, sore and worn out, feeling that his whole day had been spent in vain. Since the man was showing discouragement, the Adversary (Satan) decided to enter the picture by placing thoughts into the man's weary mind. "You have been pushing against that rock for a long time, and it hasn't moved," thus giving the man the impression that the task was impossible and that he was a failure. These thoughts discouraged and disheartened the man. "Why kill myself over this?" he thought. "I'll just put in my time, giving just the minimum effort, and that will be good enough." And that is what he planned to do until, one day, he decided to make it a matter of prayer and take his troubled thoughts to the Lord. "Lord," he said, "I have labored long and hard in Your service, putting all my strength to do that which You have asked. Yet, after all this time, I have not even budged that rock by half a millimeter. What is wrong? Why am I failing?" The Lord responded compassionately. "My son, when asked you to serve Me and you accepted, I told you that your task was to push against the rock with all of your strength, which you have done. Never once did I mention to you that I expected you to move it. Your task was [just] to push. And now you have come to Me with your strength spent, thinking that you have failed. But, is that really so? Look at yourself. Your *arms are strong and muscled, you are sinewy and brown, your hands are callused from constant pressure, your legs have become massive and hard. Through opposition, you have grown much, and your abilities now surpass that which you used to have. Yes, you haven't moved the rock. But your calling was to be obedient, to [just] push and to exercise your faith and trust in My wisdom. This you have done. Now I, My son, will move the rock." At times, when we hear a word from God, we tend to use our own intellect to decipher what He wants, when actually what God wants is just simple obedience and faith in Him. By all means, exercise the faith that moves mountains...but know that it is still God who moves mountains. When everything seems to go wrong...just P.U.S.H. When the job gets you down...just P.U.S.H. When people don't react the way you think they should... just P.U.S.H. When your money looks "gone" and the bills are due...just P.U.S.H. When people just don't understand you...just P.U.S.H.*

P = Pray

U = Until

S = Something

H =Happens

When things seem heavy for your shoulders, think of this![151]

---

[151] Anonymous author.

In my library of Living Medicine, I have memories that are stored away like my books on the shelf. I can take them out, look at them, re-experience them and then put them back. One of these memories is still very vividly etched in my mind, as if it happened yesterday.

I remember being called away from the breakfast table one morning as a nine-year-old child in India, because a snake charmer was in our front yard. He told us that he had a cobra in his basket that he had just caught and asked my father if he would like to see it. Being of a curious nature, Dad agreed, and the snake charmer told us all to stand back at least fifteen feet. The snake charmers in India use a technique of removing the fangs of the cobra to decrease the danger of working with them. This new snake had not yet had its fangs removed, so it was potentially very dangerous. The snake charmer put the basket with the cobra in front of him and, as he lifted the lid, he immediately began to play his gourd flute. As quick as a flash, the cobra traveled a good ten or fifteen feet away. As soon as the first notes came out of the flute, the cobra *immediately* stopped, raised itself up, opened its hood, turned around and came back to stop right in front of the snake charmer's knee. It continued to weave gently back and forth, as if hypnotized by the music. The snake charmer then stopped playing his flute momentarily to throw a blanket over the snake and put it back into the basket. But before he could get the blanket over the cobra, it struck and bit him on his index finger. The snake charmer did not react to being bitten by the snake and proceeded to wrap the cobra up in the blanket and place it into the basket. My father, being a physician, started to apply some emergency measures in this situation, but the snake charmer calmly said: "No, Dr. Sahib, I can take care of this myself." He then wrapped a pliable root around his upper arm as a tourniquet, reached into a little box and removed a small black object that resembled a stone. He placed it on his bitten finger, then rested that hand on his knee. *Immediately* the snake charmer developed a severe tremor in the hand that had been bitten and began to sweat profusely. After five or ten minutes, the tremor quieted down, and the black stone *eventually* dropped off his finger. He then picked up the stone and tapped it on his flute, after which several drops of yellow, viscous, sticky fluid fell on the instrument, discoloring it. My father was *so* fascinated with this whole procedure that he asked the snake charmer about the black stone. The snake charmer told him that it was the brain of a Himalayan tree frog, which had been slowly processed in heat until it became carbonized. All the snake charmers in India had been using this healing modality for centuries. He said that they also all know that, after receiving thirty-two bites from a cobra, they need to get out of the business of snake charming, because any further venom left in their system would cause chronic neurological damage. Following this discussion with my dad, the snake charmer then took the small black stone and placed it back in the little box. He told us he would boil it in milk with spices before he finally put it away for future use.

To our knowledge there has been no research done about removing snake venom in this way, yet detailed therapeutic techniques have evolved around the world to produce similar results.[152] It is interesting that the snake charmers have known since ancient times that the toxins from the snake's venom that impact the nervous system could be alleviated by using nerve tissue from another reptile. The carbonized brain of the tree frog attracts the snake venom *vibrationally* in such a way as to extract it from the nerves of the snake charmer. What is the energy that allows this "like attracts like" reality to manifest? *Energy medicine* in the form of homeopathy!

One of my other personal memories with a message for Living Medicine comes to mind when I look back to a time in November, 1982. I participated in a lecture for The American School Health Association with a Navajo Indian medicine man, a Yaqui Indian medicine man, a Vietnamese woman (whose husband was a Western physician and whose father was a traditional Vietnamese physician),

---

[152] https://www.pbs.org>wnet>the-reptiles-snakes-venomous-cures.

and our own nurse practitioner, Edna Germain. The audience consisted of some three hundred school nurses and education-related health professionals. It was an exciting morning, because we found that all five of us were basically saying the same thing. Namely, that **in any tradition, healing comes from** *within* **each individual** *and, as we all became involved in the healing arts, we* each *developed various tools that performed similar tasks. Each* one of us had had *years* of training, *years* of working within our respective cultures and *years* of developing our own respective healing arts. Each of us had been involved in successful healings through methods and modalities that, if nothing else, remained mysterious and unknown. It later occurred to me that, *in the West, we have assumed an incredible arrogance which says that the only* real *cures that work come from our own scientific model.* This kind of presumptuousness closes doors, intimidates people and can set us back in consciousness instead of allowing us to move forward.

That same week, our small *Casa Grande Dispatch* newspaper had a series of three extensive articles dealing with health care in our nation. The primary question was whether we have the moral right to decide on the use of lifesaving measures based on economics. It was interesting to me, however, that this extensive series NEVER addressed the *individual patient's right* to make this decision. The responsibility of the patients themselves for their own health care was *not even considered*, nor was the idea of "giving the body back to its rightful owner" even intimated. It failed to mention nutrition, exercise, spiritual attunement or the idea that individual people have the *right*, and *also* the responsibility, to pay attention to *their own* health care. Instead, the articles revolved around the concept that the *physician* was the one who made the decisions as to whether a person lived or died, and that this was the *physician's* responsibility. I believe that, **as physicians, we are** *not* **God and do** *not* **have the right to say whether a patient lives or dies.** However, we certainly have the *duty* to teach our patients how to take care of themselves and take responsibility for *their own* decisions, *including* their own life and death decisions. Nowhere in this extensive series, though, was it ever mentioned that *physicians* also *need to assume responsibility for* their *health choices!*

Since my library is a *living* space, it brings me right up to 2005, when I was given the opportunity to go back to the villages of North India and Afghanistan for three months. In India, I had the privilege of conducting physical exams and nutritional assessments for nearly nine hundred children in the children's home that my parents and my Aunt Belle (Lorena Belle Taylor, DO) had started in the late 1940's to care for the children of leper parents. These are wonderful children who need all the help they can get, since leprosy remains a huge problem in India to this day, despite medication and great strides that have been made to control it. From India, I went to Afghanistan to work with my brother (Carl) and Shukria Hussan, MD under the auspices of the Future Generations[153] organization. Since Afghanistan has been a war-torn country since the 1970's, women and children have *especially* suffered under these circumstances. *At that time, the maternal mortality rate was higher in Afghanistan than in* any other *place in the world.* It was my prayer that I might be able to help.

We knew it was important for us to be able to talk to older women who had experienced *multiple* pregnancies to get some idea of why conditions were so bad. To do this, we had to first get permission from the *men* in the villages, who initially said no. They only agreed when Dr. Hussan told the men that the women we wanted to interview were their mothers-in-law! Once the men agreed to *that*, we were able to set up week-long programs where we lived with these women in a secluded place. We had asked for two women from ten different small villages in the Bamiyan district of Afghanistan, as we thought we could handle twenty women very well in the house we had rented. To our great surprise, *fifty* women showed up! We had to send twenty of them back, since thirty was the absolute

[153] www.future.org

maximum number we could work with in that space. Some of these women brought their small children along with them, even their nursing babies. *They had* all *had between two and fourteen pregnancies.* Most of them had lost from one to six children, and all of them had stories of deep suffering and pain. Each told us *her story* of *each* pregnancy, birth and postpartum course. These stories brought to light some very interesting facts:

- *The Afghani people had NO understanding of the anatomy and physiology of pregnancy and labor.* They understood *how* women got pregnant, though *what happened after that was a major mystery* to men and women alike! They thought it was some miraculous process that kind of took care of itself. Because of this *extreme* lack of knowledge, it seemed important that Dr. Hussan and I take the time to explain to the women *in detail* what was *really* happening to their bodies. So, with my one piece of chalk and a small blackboard, I began sketching the anatomy of the reproductive system, and they became excited. I drew a picture of the vagina and cervix, as well as the fallopian tubes and ovaries. I explained to the women how the egg grew in the ovaries and was then transported down the fallopian tubes into the uterus, implanting itself in the wall of the uterus after it was impregnated by the sperm. The idea that the uterus was actually a muscular structure which contracted like other muscles to allow the baby to be born was fascinating to them. I also explained that the sperm had traveled up the vagina and into the uterus and then swam up into the fallopian tube to meet the egg. I told them that, when the egg and sperm got together, the cells began to divide and then the baby began to grow and develop in the uterus in their abdomen until it was ready to be born. I emphasized to them how important it was for the cervix to fully open up *before* the baby could come through and be born. This information was very fascinating and exciting to these women. One woman asked me how many sperm got deposited into the vagina. I told her *millions!* She then asked: "How many eggs?" I said: "One—and THAT egg gets to choose which sperm it wants!" With that *one* bit of information, these women put their shoulders back and held their heads up high—*it was the* first *time in their lives that they realized they had any choice about what went on in their lives and within their bodies!* This knowledge boosted their self-esteem, self-respect and strength. They were ecstatic and Dr. Hussan and I were in tears.

• The reason this basic anatomy and physiology lesson was so important was because *the Afghani people had NO IDEA how to get the baby out of the mother if the mother did not have enough strength to push the baby out herself.* This meant someone from the outside had to help her. The only way they knew to do that was to put pressure on the mother's abdomen from the outside. If the husband was around and was strong enough, then he would be the one who would push from above the uterus down towards the perineum. This action, of course, frequently resulted in the death of the mother or the baby. Even if the birth *was* accomplished, it was frequently accompanied by severe tissue damage, including a ruptured uterus and/or bladder, a torn perineum, recto-vaginal fissures and/or severe incontinence, representing the *major* causes of maternal mortality among these women. If these complications of pregnancy did not *kill* the mother, they could render the woman a *total* social outcast for the *rest of her life*, as well as subject her to infections and multiple pelvic diseases. The whole birthing process for these women was truly like "going through the valley of the shadow of death." This scenario is all that these wonderfully strong women knew and expected, yet were willing to go through to birth a baby. Dr. Hussan and I felt both horrified and in awe as we listened to these women's stories.

- When a woman found out she was pregnant, there were *certain food taboos that prevented her from eating "cold foods" throughout the pregnancy*, especially calcium-rich foods (milk, eggs, yogurt, carrots, etc.). Almost all these women said they had muscle spasms when they went into labor, which I believe was actually hypocalcemic tetany.

- *When a woman went into labor, she was not given anything to eat or drink until the baby was born.*

- *The birth usually took place directly on a dirt floor assisted by someone who had no training or understanding of the birthing process and/or hygiene.*

These Afghani women were anxious to learn, and hungrily soaked up the information we gave them. We had a wonderful time. In the middle of the week, some of the women got up and began dancing. I took pictures of them and, when I showed them to some staff people of Future Generations, the men said: "Don't let their husbands see those pictures, because *women aren't supposed to dance, laugh or have fun.* If their husbands see these pictures, they'll be severely punished."

I heard from my brother (Carl) and Dr. Hussan that a *follow-up meeting* with these women occurred *a month after we had been there.* The news was very exciting. Twenty-eight of the thirty women came back. They all said that as soon as they returned to their villages, they spent four days in the mosque with the other village women. The women who had *not* been able to participate in the workshop came to *these* women with whom we had spent the week, asking them what they had learned and how they could work together in *their* villages also. *This is a perfect example of the Physician Within each of the women* Dr. Hussan and I had met with *sharing* their *knowledge with the Physician Within each of the* other *women* in the villages who did not attend our workshop. In that way, the women who did not attend the workshop could benefit as well from the new information we had imparted. *None* of these Afghani women had any educational degrees that qualified them to do this! They reported that births had been successfully performed without starving the women, and they had begun utilizing clean cloths for the births and clean/proper cord-cutting procedures. Prior to our visit, the women had used *any* instrument available (including a stone) to cut the cord. That practice had resulted in neonatal tetanus, which, of course, is one of the diseases that causes infant death. The women also said that they had done a lot to improve their hygienic conditions, as well as their nutritional status. Efforts to help these Afghani women continue to this day through the work of Future Generations, as *women teach other women* what they have learned. In addition, the Afghani health system has established a program to train midwives, who are primarily young girls between the ages of sixteen and twenty. Unfortunately, this midwifery training program has *not* been very successful. This seems to be due to the fact that, *once trained*, most of these young girls are *no longer interested in going back to live in their remote villages* and doing this type of work. They prefer working in the towns, cities and hospitals that offer better working and lifestyle conditions. This experience was a rich and rewarding one for me, and I have many precious memories of these beautiful people. *They continue to teach each other as they continue to learn*, building their own Living Medicine library of knowledge and experiences.

In addition to our physical library shelves, each of us has within our psyche our own *personal* library where we have stored our experiences. This memory bank offers us a place where we can access information, which helps us continue to live and grow. As physicians, our libraries also allow us to share in the knowledge and healing aspects of the *past* as we evolve the healing techniques and concepts for the future. For example, the computer has now brought to our fingertips the availability of information and therapies that have *never* been *readily* accessible to us before. Within moments, we can access the available therapies for *any* specific disease process and see how they interact with other therapeutic modalities. We can access the patient's medical history, all their medications and even their latest vital signs, through these electronic records. Amazing amounts of information, from the widely known to the obscure, become available to us, and we need to learn to use this technology *effectively* in our practices.

As previously discussed at length in chapter two, in *my* lifetime the *science* of medicine has advanced so far that it is truly amazing. Our challenge *now* is to take this incredible scientific information and *infuse it with Life*, so that it can *truly* be used to help us practice more effectively the *art* of medicine *along with* the science. *It is our job as physicians to help the patient use* any and all *available knowledge to assist them in their healing process.* We need to support them to *not* be overwhelmed or terrified by so much information. **Scientific information is such an awesome tool, and we need to constantly be learning how to *apply it in the best way possible* to further the *art* of medicine**. The following explanation of how we came to be using *cell-signaling formulas* to support our immune systems during the COVID-19 pandemic is worth sharing at this point. It is just *one example* of the kind of collaboration that Dr. Ann and I both are *currently* experiencing firsthand that has moved its holistic approach into the Living Medicine paradigm by infusing it with Life and living.

The originator of the *isoenergetic cell-signaling*™ approach to healing was Barbara A. Brewitt, PhD, MDiv (1948-2009). Through her doctoral research in biological structure at the University of Washington School of Medicine in 1989, as well as her postdoctoral studies as a National Institutes of Health (NIH) Fellow, Barbara became recognized as *an international expert on cell-to-cell communication*. As a result of her contributions, she broadened our understanding that ***growth factors*** (a type of cell signal) ***are related to health and healing***. Her research was so successful that it was translated into eight languages. Like all pioneers, however, Barbara was maligned by some colleagues who did not *fully* comprehend her research and attempted to discredit both her and her work. Nevertheless, by combining the principles of *molecular biology* and *biophysics* with those gleaned from *homeopathy* over a two-hundred-fifty-year period, Barbara and Paul Opheim (her research associate) created nine different cell-signaling formulas that were *safe, clinically-proven* and have stood the test of time. Their first *double-blind, placebo-controlled clinical study*, published in 1995, proved that a set of particular non-molecular isopathic growth factors could prevent HIV-positive adults from losing lean body mass and experiencing opportunistic infections over a six-month period. Two other research studies showed equally impressive clinical outcomes. All of their studies were *peer-reviewed* and published in the medical literature, qualifying their formulas as "evidence-based" medicine. Multiple *proof-of-hypothesis case studies* conducted since 1995, as well as *hundreds of anecdotal reports* from medical practitioners around the world, have *repeatedly validated* the effectiveness of their formulas. Subsequent to Barbara's untimely death in 2009, Paul has researched and developed many other medicinal formulas for both chronic and acute conditions (see complete list on his website).[154]

Dr. Ann has been aware of these cell-signaling medicines for over twenty-five years. She was introduced to them by Barbara in her Seattle, Washington practice to use as part of her treatment protocol with HIV patients. After Barbara died in 2009, Dr. Ann thought the formulas were no longer available. She was unable to include them as part of her overall treatment approach again until the fall of 2019, when she met Paul for the first time. Since then, she has been able to reintroduce this *highly effective holistic medical therapy* back into her practice. She uses these formulas in

---

[154] www.LepticaMedical.com – access is user-name and password-restricted for physicians.

conjunction with all her other therapeutic modalities to help her patients reach their treatment goals sooner and more cost-effectively. She and Paul are also currently co-conducting *two small clinical trials with veterans* at the Warrior Healing Center in Sierra Vista, Arizona using the PTSD formula as well as his recently-developed formulas for COVID-19 immune support. Their collaborative "white paper" (research document) is posted on both of their websites. It describes in detail the preliminary results of their PTSD study (which are *extremely* promising), as well as Paul's *thorough* discussion of the *science* behind his COVID-19 *immune support* formulas (*way above* both of our heads!). Their collaboration is one of the best *current* examples of Living Medicine in action: combining the *best* of both the art *and* science of medicine to solve a problem *not* focused on the killing that is challenging the very existence of Life itself in 2020. Instead, this *unique* "do no harm" approach is infused with Life and living. It stands in stark contrast to the other conventional,[155] alternative,[156,157] complementary[158,159,160] and holistic[161] medicine approaches that *all have valid research* behind them to show that they work to *kill* COVID-19, either directly or indirectly. We find it especially ironic, however, that these *science-based* approaches are *all* being maligned and devalued, and their

---

[155] https://covid19criticalcare.com.

[156] https://aepromo.org/en/ozonized-saline-solution-o3ss-could-be-an-effective-supplement-in-the-management-of-patients-with-covid-19/?inf_contact_key=95cc66d10b3d05e5ac3dde105601fb3b.

[157] Stone, Will. "Using UV Light to Fight COVID-19 Spread" www.medscape.com (July 23, 2020).

[158] https://articles.mercola.com/sites/articles/archive/2020/04/20/zinc-dosage-for-immune-system.aspx?cid_medium=etaf&cid=share

[159] Risch, Harvey A., MD, PhD. https://www.newsweek.com/key-defeating-covid-19-already-exists-we-need-start-using-it-opinion-1519535 (7-23-20).

[160] Risch, Harvey A., MD, PhD. https://academic.oup.com>early-outpatient-treatment-of-symptomatic-high-risk-covid-19-patients-that-should-be-ramped-up-immediately-as-key-to-the-pandemic-crisis (5-27-20).

[161] Brownstein, David, MD et.al. "A Novel Approach to Treating COVID-19 Using Nutritional and Oxidative Therapies," Science, Public Health Policy and the Law, Vol 2:4-22 (July 2020), Clinical and Translational Research (IPAK PHPI).

efficacy superseded by politics and greed; *not unlike* science *has done to the* art *of medicine for many decades* now. In the throes of this 2020 pandemic, Living Medicine is needed now *more than ever*, and is truly *a paradigm whose time has* more than *come*.

6

The Bedroom

A central room in our house of Living Medicine is the bedroom. Whether situated in a two-million-dollar mansion or a mud hut, the bedroom is the place where only *selected* people are invited in. It is the place where the most intimate relationships are shared and where the most profound personal experiences take place. We retire to our bedroom when it is time for us to move into that aspect of our life that our conscious and unconscious minds share. Most of us, in an average day, spend about a third of our time in our bedroom. It truly is a "holy of holies." Many of us even have a small personal altar in our bedroom. Our bedroom furniture, whether it is an engraved canopy bed or a bedding roll, is our own personal furniture. This room is truly meant to be *our safe place,* and, when we are sick, this is the room where we prefer to go.

One very important role of the bedroom is that it is the place for rest. When it is time for sleep, we retire to our bedroom. Over the years, I have heard many complaints about sleep from my patients. They say things like: "It's three o'clock in the morning. I feel like I haven't slept a wink, and I have a day that's going to be busy and active. What do I do?" Sleep is so wonderful, so refreshing and so important; and *like* clean *air,* clean *water and* clean *food, we all need sleep to live.* "And yet we are a sleep-sick society, ignorant of the facts of sleep—and the price of sleep deprivation," writes William C.

Dement, MD, PhD.[162] As the world's leading authority on sleep, sleep deprivation and the diagnosis and treatment of sleep disorders, Dr. Dement's research has empirically proven that *"healthful sleep...is... more influential than diet, exercise or heredity...in predicting longevity."* In his opinion, "the price we have paid for ignoring sleep...is an epidemic of heart disease...[as well as] immeasurable mental and psychological disadvantages." His research also shows that thirty-three percent of all traffic accidents are fatigue-related.

Of all the complaints I have heard from patients through the years, *insomnia* seems to be one of the most frequent. I believe the most important thing in dealing with insomnia has to do with our *attitude* and accepting ourselves where we are with respect to our own individual, very personal, sleep patterns and needs. It is also important to remember that, *as we age, our sleep patterns change*, and eight hours of sleep may *not* be as essential as it was when we were younger. As older adults, even when we have interrupted sleep, we still can awaken refreshed with an adequate night's rest. Personally, I find that I might need more than eight hours of sleep on some days; on other days, I might need less than that. At this stage of my life, I really need an afternoon nap *every* day! I find that my sleep and rest needs vary from day to day, depending on how I feel and what is going on in my life. In addition, I also find that those of us who are older can get away with what I call "good downtime." This means that I am in bed and resting. I may or may *not* be dozing—my body is functioning and comfortable—I am just not asleep. During this time, I try to let my mind reminisce on the good things in my life instead of the problematic ones. I also try to take this time to let my mind reach out to those I love on this plane or any other plane. I also say some prayers of gratitude and pray for everybody I can think of who is in my life, now or in the past. I try to think about the beauty I have experienced during my long life. If I can do this, I find that not only does time go faster while I am in

---

[162] Dement, William C. MD, PhD and Christopher Vaughan. The Promise of Sleep: A Pioneer in Sleep Medicine Explores the Vital Connection Between Health, Happiness and a Good Night's Sleep, 2000.

bed, I also sometimes fall asleep! Even if I do *not* fall asleep, I find my-self refreshed and joyful when I get up, as eight hours of "good down-time" *can be* regenerating and energy-replenishing. If I start worrying about something, however, and begin to fret (or find myself feeling angry, frustrated or anxious), I not only do not rest, I wake up feeling fatigued and irritable. *This is* particularly *true if I start worrying about* not *sleeping!* When I put my energy into the idea that I am in bed and am supposed to be asleep, yet I am *not* sleeping, all I find myself do-ing is building up more and more anxiety. The more this happens, the less I sleep. The less I sleep, the more anxious I feel, and I go 'round and 'round on that merry-go-round and find it difficult to step off. The most important thing to remember, though, is this: **as physicians, if we listen to our patients carefully and compassionately, we can sometimes find a clue to their insomnia.** By doing this, we can **help them deal with the *underlying* issue**, which would be *far* more helpful than prescribing a sleeping pill and them having to live with its side effects!

For some of my patients, when they cannot sleep, it is helpful to get up and fix a cup of tea, or get up and read something relax-ing, and then go back to bed. Watching TV (especially the news or a scary movie) or reading a murder mystery *rarely* offers any help in getting to sleep. In addition, it is best not to eat a heavy meal before going to bed, as *the activity of the intestinal tract at bedtime can be disconcerting and cause sleeplessness.* Remember, too, that having a digital clock or other electrical equipment (such as TV's, comput-ers and cell phones) in the bedroom, *especially* anywhere close to the bed, creates an electrical field around the body that can make it difficult sleep.[163,164] For that reason, it is recommended to turn off *all* electrical equipment in the bedroom when you are ready to go to sleep, *in addition to unplugging it.* Move your digital clock at least ten

---

[163] Becker, Robert O. Cross Currents: The Perils of Electropollution, The Promise of Electromedicine, 1990.

[164] Milham, Samuel, MD, MPH. Dirty Electricity: Electrification and the Diseases of Civilization, 2012.

feet away from your bed. Lastly, look outside your window. Are there high-tension wires, cell phone towers, or worse—5G technologies, near your home? These can also wreak havoc with your nervous system, making it difficult to sleep as well as function optimally when you are awake.[165,166,167] It is best to *do all you can to make your bedroom a comfortable, pleasant place where you like to spend time, and you will be more apt to have a restful sleep.* Protecting yourself from these harmful technological influences when you are out and about, as well as when you are at home, will also promote more restful sleep. In addition, some people find *personal sleep trackers*[168,169] to be helpful, which come in both wearable and non-wearable forms. Though not as accurate as a *professional sleep study* (conducted at home or in an overnight clinical setting to evaluate *serious* sleep disorders like sleep apnea), these trackers can often give useful clues about the *quality* of your sleep, so that you can take steps to improve it.

Sleep is not the only thing our bedrooms are used for. My last two children were born in my bedroom. It is where I rocked my children to sleep and nursed them when they were tiny. It is where they jumped on our bed to awaken us and romp with us in the morning. It is where my husband and I spent our own private time together. It is probably the place where the tenderest of all emotions and feelings are shared. Where else can we have a good cry or laugh until we cannot even sit up? For many people, the bedroom is the most comfortable place for us when we die.

Living Medicine involves the very act of giving and receiving from the *conscious to the unconscious* parts of ourselves as well as from those parts of ourselves to other people. *One without the other is not complete*. This principle is manifested in *every*

---

[165] Pineault, Nicolas. The Non-Tinfoil Guide to EMF's, 2017.

[166] Mercola, Joseph, DO. EMF*D: 5G, Wi-Fi & Cell Phone – Hidden Harms and How to Protect Yourself, 2020.

[167] http://earthcalm.com/

[168] www.nosleeplessnights.com>best-sleep-trackers-in-2020-reviewed-and-compared.

[169] www.wareable.com>health-and-wellbeing-best-sleep-trackers.

breath we take. We release the carbon dioxide used by plants, and we take in the oxygen that plants produce. Birth and death are like that. The woman releases the egg from the ovary, so that the sperm released by the male can be taken into the egg. The egg is now no longer *just* an egg. *Together* with the sperm, it becomes an embryo. The embryo must then be willing to let go of old patterns and develop new ones. If at any place along the way it decides to keep the old patterns and *not* shift into the new ones, it dies. One statement from the Cayce material reads: "Ovulation is the law of nature. Conception is the law of God."[170] *To grow and develop into a human child, the embryo has to be constantly* willing, *on a molecular level,* to change in order to live.

When the time comes for the baby to be born, there must be a letting go of the comfort and security of the womb, which was its bedroom prior to birth. The baby then comes out into the world, where s/he will have to breathe and eat and get rid of waste on its own. *No longer can the mother do this for the baby.* For the rest of the baby's life, s/he must be willing to give and receive on *all* levels—physically, mentally, emotionally and spiritually. Only as babies are willing to do this will they continue to grow. Throughout life, we breathe in and out, food goes in and out, muscles contract and relax. When all this activity stops, we die. It is then that we release the physical, so that the soul can continue its journey.

Metaphorically, it is not a far stretch to think of the uterus as the bedroom of a baby while preparing for birth. We now know that many babies can hear and feel what is going on in the life of the mother,[171,172,173] just as we, in our bedrooms, know what is going on in the rest of the house. In the work that I have done with newborns, it

---

[170] www.edgarcayce.org. Reading 457-11.

[171] Gabriel, Michael. *Voices from the Womb: Consciousness and Trauma in the Pre-Birth Self,* 1992.

[172] David Chamberlain, PhD. *Windows to the Womb: Revealing the Conscious Baby from Conception to Birth,* 2013.

[173] Susan Highsmith, PhD. *The Renaissance of Birth: Changing the Language of Childbirth,* 2014.

has also become ever clearer to me that *the attitudes and emotions of the people surrounding the baby at birth are* indelibly *etched into his/her soul pattern.* Having just been removed from the secure environment of the uterus where everything was provided, the baby now must learn to deal with *other* people's emotions on their own.

When we were in England with an A.R.E. group led by Hugh Lynn Cayce in 1969, a psychic by the name of Ronald Beasley spoke to us. He drew a picture of the auras (the body's energy *fields*) surrounding different people. Some individuals had an aura forming *smoothly* at the top, while others had an aura that were *twisted* at the top. I asked Ronald: "Why the difference?" His response was that the ones whose auras were twisted were the people whose souls had not been properly tucked in with care when they were born. *To me, this was a pivotal concept.* I truly believe the emotions and thoughts of those present with us at birth and death impact the type of experience the soul making these transitions will experience. **If, when a baby is born, there is joy and jubilation, that soul enters this earth with a feeling of being accepted and wanted. If, on the other hand, the baby is greeted with negative emotion, that soul will feel unwanted and rejected.** *This can cause confusion and trauma, which that soul may struggle with all its life.* The following story demonstrates the *profound* impact of this concept in one person's life.

I had a patient who was in her mid-fifties and the third child in a family in which the first two siblings were boys. When she was born, her father was unable to make it to the hospital. Even if he *had* been there, he would not have been allowed in the delivery room. When he did arrive at the hospital, the nurse informed him that he had a baby girl. His response was: "That's not possible. We don't have girls in our family." *He said it as a joke, yet he insisted that the nurse remove the baby's diaper so he could be sure that she was a girl and not a boy.* Every year on her birthday, he repeated this story, because he thought it was funny. He *consciously* did no harm, and not only did he *not* reject his daughter throughout her life, he adored her (and she, him). However, *as a newborn,* my patient felt that her father not only rejected her as a person, he also rejected her gender and who she was as she came to this earth. This experience at birth (and being reminded of it *every* year on her birthday) caused problems for her during her *entire* life. It affected *all* her relationships and also her own acceptance of who she was as a female child and as an adult woman. It was clearly apparent to me that rejecting her gender caused my patient deep trauma. Fortunately, she understood this and realized she needed counseling. *She worked to heal that trauma* all *her life*. Others who have been either rejected or traumatized at birth may or may not know that *such rejection leaves deep scars*. Fortunately, emotional pain like this can often be dealt with by using techniques like rebirthing.

Another example of the impact of this kind of rejection at birth happened to a friend of mine who has struggled her whole life with feelings of insecurity and still lacks a strong sense of personhood. She told me that when she was born, she was very thin and wrinkled. Perceiving her child as ugly, her mother covered her daughter up with a small towel when anybody came to visit. This behavior went on for many months and became the "family joke" through the years. People laughed about this story and thought it was very funny. The reality, though, is that this newborn little girl was traumatized by her mother's actions. She was further traumatized by the persistent, repeated telling of this "funny" story. She *continues* to feel rejected and unable to truly appreciate her own beauty despite the fact that she is *now* an attractive seventy-year-old woman who has had a successful career as a counselor in the local high school.

These two examples demonstrate how deeply this type of trauma to a person's psyche surrounding their birth can have *life-long effects*. **As Living Medicine physicians, we *truly* need to listen to our patients' life stories, carefully and compassionately, in order to find the *root cause* of some of their problems.** Stephen Covey[174] summed up the process that it takes to do this as follows (paraphrase and bold is mine):

---

[174] Covey, Stephen. *The 7 Habits of Highly Effective People*, 1989.

...if we want to make relatively minor changes in our [patients'] *lives, we can perhaps appropriately focus on* [their] *attitudes and behaviors. But if we want to make significant, quantum change, we need to work on* [their] *basic paradigms. In the words of Thoreau: "For every thousand hacking at the leaves of evil, there is one striking at the root." We can only achieve quantum improvements in our* [patients'] *lives as we quit hacking at the leaves of attitude and behavior and get to work on the root* [causes], *the paradigms from which* [**all**] *attitudes and behaviors flow.*

Just like the previous two stories illustrate the negative impact that events during birthing can cause, there are also *favorable outcomes* that can occur from a *positive birthing experience*, as the following story illustrates.

My daughter (Helene)'s youngest son (Andrew) was born in her bedroom, and I had the privilege of helping her birth him. The people in attendance were her husband (Fred) and our Navajo nurse, Ernestine. Ernestine had had three children of her own, though she had never been involved in a birthing for another woman. Things were going along quite well until the contractions became severe, and Helene was in hard labor. Suddenly, Ernestine began jumping up and down around the room and waving her hands. I said: "What in the world are you doing?" She said: "Navajo blessing! Navajo blessing!" and continued until she was through with her Navajo blessing. This blessing is a tradition in her culture and is used to assist both the pregnant mother and her baby to have a good outcome during the birthing process,[175] which can often be a stressful time for both. I know that this activity in that bedroom helped both Helene and her newborn son that day, and it was certainly part of the sacred experience that the rest of us

---

[175] Lang, R. Blessingway into Birth: A Rite of Passage, 1993.

shared. I also believe that the Navajo blessing Andrew received from Ernestine at birth influenced him for the rest of his life. As a result, he grew up to become a physician who will begin his ER residency training in 2020, a career which will give *him* the opportunity to help people during stressful times.

During the birthing of a baby, if our whole focus is on *killing*— even killing the pain of childbirth—**we may even** *accentuate* **the pain by centering our attention on it.** *When we try to hang on to something that no longer serves its purpose, we create a block that results in pain.* I have worked many hours with my obstetrics patients by having them move into the pain of the contraction, breathing and relaxing with it, *instead of* tightening up against it or fighting it. We can use music or color, or their partner's hands, to apply pressure in the area where the pain remains greatest. The mother can also shift her pelvis into a more *effective* position to help reduce her pain, which will also help her baby to move down and out. Sometimes a chant helps— anything *that allows her to participate in the whole process, rather than trying to escape from it.* When a woman can do this, she needs *less* pain medicine and intervention. If she rides the wave of her pain like a surfer rides the ocean waves, she will move *with* the energy of Life and Love. *It is when we fight against the movement of Life that pain becomes more severe.* The fact of the matter is that women generally deal quite well with pain most of the time during labor. What they do *not* manage well is fear and abandonment. **If a woman has support during labor, she can handle the pain much better than if she feels alone and abandoned.** Much like the children in the previous examples who experienced traumatic births, *mothers can also be traumatized* by a lack of support during this most sacred time. Some of them, *like the children of traumatic births*, are affected by this trauma *for the rest of their lives.* I have often wondered to what degree such trauma plays a part in postpartum depression.

During the years I was doing home births with Barbara Brown, a nurse practitioner and midwife, we created the "Baby Buggy" program. It was in the 1950's when women were beginning to want to have their babies born at home. We had a mobile unit that one of us would drive to the home of the mother in labor, so that we could have any equipment that might be needed for the birth readily available, including IV solutions. It was also equipped with emergency supplies in the event we needed to transport the mother and baby to the hospital.

During one of these home births, Barbara worked with a young woman who had been involved in a religious group in which meditation played a central role. Therefore, she not only knew how to meditate, she had spent many hours doing so. However, she had not really accepted the fact that there might be pain and discomfort associated with her labor. She became more and more distraught, because she felt like she could not get herself into the meditative state she had been counting on to get her through the birth. Throughout this time the cervix was not dilating. It stayed at one centimeter and, for several hours, she remained in good hard labor with no progress whatsoever. Finally, Barbara remembered the patient's previous experience with meditation and recalled that she knew how to chant. Barbara realized that if this woman could come up with a chant that would work for her, then maybe she could move past the block that her pain was causing and get on with the birth. So, Barbara said: "Now dear, I want you to start chanting "open lotus, lotus open, open lotus, lotus open." The young woman immediately knew how to do this and began chanting. Within a few hours, the cervix opened to complete dilatation! Now it was time to push. However, the patient was not *emotionally* ready to push. Trying to help, Barbara suggested that pushing the baby out was like having a large bowel movement. This young woman did not want her baby to be compared to a bowel movement! Barbara recognized that she needed another chant. The chant that she came up with was "down and out, down and out." With this chant, the young woman was able to push and birthed her baby spontaneously!

For millennia, women have worked with other women in the birthing process. They have even created a birthing dance called the "belly dance."[176] Women did this dance throughout their pregnancy to keep the pelvis mobile and alive, so that the baby did not get stuck in one position and need to be pushed out or extracted. There were certain dance positions and movements that helped the process. For example, during labor, women would dance around the birthing mother as she participated in the dance as best she could.

When men became obstetricians, they felt it was their duty to help "stop the pain," so *medications were introduced.* The whole birthing process then became something to fight *against*, to "rescue" women from their pain. *They thought the mother did not feel the pain, if medicated.* In reality, women DO feel their labor pains! Medication sometimes just dulls their memory of them. Far worse, however, is the fact that **medications administered during labor often do *not* allow women to work with their pain effectively.** One of the side effects of these medications can be that *the mother may not even know for many hours that her baby has been born*—or, worse, have a lack of memory of the birth all together. Sometimes these medications create hallucinatory experiences for the mother that take her completely out of her birthing process. I did not know I had a son with my first birth until twenty-four hours after he was born. Even then, I was too groggy to really respond and bond with him. Also, when women are medicated during labor, the action of fighting against the pain causes *fear* to be the dominant emotion surrounding the birth. Muscles tighten, and the women feel alone in "the valley of the shadow of death." *Babies born this way experience more trauma themselves, as do their mothers.* Sometimes, when these children are told the details about their birth later in life, they feel guilty for "causing" their mothers so much pain. These examples, of course, do *not* mean that there are not times when **surgery and medication** are needed. I believe, though, that the use of these modalities **should be the EXCEPTION and *not* the rule, and** thus be **used only on a *case-by-case basis*, with caution and as a *last* resort.**

---

[176] Zimmerman, Rachel. "New Labor Moves: Belly Dancing Hits Delivery Room, www.wsj.com (August 4, 2007).

The whole process of labor remains mysterious for many people. As explained in detail in the last chapter, my trip to Afghanistan helped me realize that these wonderful Afghani women really knew *nothing* about this process. They had no idea what was in their unborn baby's bedroom. As difficult as these facts were to hear and deal with regarding the Afghani women's circumstances, I was also horrified when I came back to the U.S. when a physician friend told me that the *caesarian section rate was up to thirty-seven percent* of *all* births in Arizona in 2006! When I heard this, I realized that what we were doing in Arizona was essentially the same as what the Afghani women were doing: using *external* means to extract the baby. The difference is that, with caesarian sections, many times it represents a matter of *convenience* instead of necessity. The Afghani women used external means because they were ignorant of the physical aspect of birthing a baby. *We* are using external means, I believe, because **we physicians are ignorant of the emotional *and* spiritual aspects of birthing a baby**. *This ignorance*, I am convinced, *is causing problems that we do not even comprehend* at this point. The difference between what *we* do and the way the Afghani women give birth is that *we can sew the tissues back together again, and they cannot.* We may think that the Afghani way of birthing is terrible. Yet, given the fact that in our country *many times caesarian sections are used for* convenience *only*, who are we to judge when ignorance is causing intervention?

On the weekend of November 10, 2006, there was a conference in Mesa, Arizona entitled "The Baby Summit." This gathering was the work of the Association of Prenatal and Perinatal Psychology and Health (APPPAH) organization, which deals with issues regarding pregnancy and birth.[177] I have known about the work of this organization for many years and regard it highly. Since I was one of the keynote speakers, I had the opportunity to talk to the whole group, addressing my concerns about the problems the women in Afghanistan were having. I mentioned the work that I had done in Tibet in 1990 with Future Generations, as well as my own work here in the United

---

[177] www.apppah.org

States. I commented that I was horrified to learn that our hospital Cae-sarian section rate in *Arizona* was *thirty-seven percent* and that most of these procedures were *elective*. A woman in the audience stood up during the question-and-answer period. She was from *Mexico* where *eighty-five percent* of the hospital deliveries are C-sections. Another woman from *Brazil* said her country's hospital delivery rate for C-sections was *ninety percent*. Much to my horror, a woman from *Iran* said that their C-section rate in hospitals was *one hundred percent!* I was appalled hearing these statistics, as were most of the people in attendance. I could hardly comprehend this information. Every rea-son for this that I could come up with made no sense. *The underlying cause must be that we, as women, have lost our sense of reality.* We know how to *have* babies. We are *built* to have babies. *We need to trust ourselves and our own bodies in the birthing process. All* babies know how to come into this world. That has been true since the begin-ning of time. Why we *now* think intervention is needed to this extent is unreal. *C-sections are* not *without their complications*, and I am aware that, *sometimes*, this procedure is indicated. However, that fact is *probably* true *only in about five percent of all births.*

Another lecture at that Baby Summit featured Joel M. Evans, MD, founder and director for The Center for Women's Health in Darien, Connecticut, assistant clinical professor at Albert Einstein College of Medicine and senior faculty at The Center for Mind-Body Medicine in Washington, D.C. He outlined *multiple* complications of C-sections. I thought to myself: *with all these known risks, why in the world would a woman choose a C-section that wasn't necessary rather than a nor-mal vaginal delivery?*

Everything the mother thinks and feels directly affects the baby. People who have been hypnotically regressed to life in the uterus can tell many stories of things that happened during their intra-uterine life. **The baby is a conscious living being, and the uterus itself responds to the mother's emotions.** The placenta knows its work and does it very well. A perfect example of this happened when a pregnant patient came in to see me (long after I had stopped birthing babies) because she had questions about her pregnancy. At seven months, she began to spot and was told that she had a "placenta previa." This meant that the placenta was covering the cervix (mouth or opening) of the uterus and that, in order to deliver the baby, she would most likely need a C-section. She had been told to go home and get off her feet. I added two recommendations. First, I suggested she use a castor oil pack over her lower abdomen—*without* heat —for as long as she was comfortable. Second, I suggested she visualize the placenta moving off of the cervix and up onto the uterine wall. I informed her that the placenta *does* move and travel throughout the inner wall of the uterus, so I suggested that she consciously visualize this happening while resting in bed. *She began doing what I prescribed, and the bleeding stopped*. When the ultrasound was repeated a month later, the placenta had moved *completely* off of the cervix and up onto the uterine wall! She carried the baby to full-term and vaginally birthed a healthy, ten-pound, redheaded, little boy!

To illustrate the eternal beauty of the magnificent structure of the pregnant uterus, I want to share with you a conversation I had with the actress Lindsay Wagner. She had just returned from attending a class with her son (Dorian) given by her childbirth instructor for children who were expecting a new brother or sister in their family. The class used charts, pictures and diagrams of the developing pregnancy, from the perspective of *both* someone on the outside watching *and* from the baby developing on the inside. Among the illustrations was a picture of the umbilical cord attached to the baby in utero from its origin in the placenta. When Dorian saw this, he said: "That looks like a tree." As Lindsay thought about this, she realized that it did indeed resemble a tree—a truly universal symbol. Every single one of us born into this dimension (the energy field into which Life manifests itself) has spent close to nine months in the uterus. As a developing fetus, there is nothing to perceive except the walls of the womb, its own hands and feet and this amazing structure from which it receives nourishment and a great deal of other information. The structure itself *is* like a tree: the placenta is its roots, the cord is its trunk and the developing baby is its limbs and fruit. The more I thought about it, the more it seemed to me that we have a wonderful opportunity to look at this symbol as the Tree of Life. From ancient times, this Tree of Life has had its roots deep in the ground and its limbs reaching up to the heavens. Its fruit grows gradually, ripens and then, much like the story of pregnancy and birth, drops to the ground to start the whole cycle all over again.

We need to understand the continuity of Life and the importance of nourishment that comes *both* from the mother to the baby *and* from the Divine to the baby via the Spark of Life. It is interesting that God is referred to as Our Father in Heaven and the earth as Mother Earth. *We are the children of this symbolic union of Spirit and flesh.* The Tree of Life then brings nourishment, *both* from the earth *and* from the heavens. The heavens give Life itself to the developing child, the fruit of the union of the sperm and the ovum. From the earth, the child is nourished with oxygen, food, minerals and all that it needs to grow. If the soil is poor, the tree does not develop well and can become sick. Good soil, on the other hand, creates health. Likewise, a baby grow-ing in the womb with a placenta *actively* bringing nutrients to it either grows in health and vigor *or* it can become ill. Physically, *the baby's health, or lack thereof, depends on the* quality *of the food the mother eats, the water she drinks and the air she breathes.* It is the *Spirit* that influences the thoughts the mother thinks, the movies she watches, the emotions she feels, the joy she expresses, as well as whatever she experiences during the pregnancy, including hope, love, faith and gentleness. *All these thoughts and feelings become part of what the baby lives with and grows with throughout the pregnancy.* If the moth-er is angry, afraid, jealous or subjected to other negative emotions or experiences, the baby derives its nourishment from *that* environment, and the Tree of Life can be blighted. *It is exciting to consider the won-derful opportunity that any mother has to nourish her baby in the way that God nourishes us.* During pregnancy, what you *eat,* what you *think* and what you *pray for* ALL become part of the consciousness of the growing fetus. By the same token, we must also remember that the *soul* of the fetus has a life plan of its own. Even though we do not really know what its life plan is, we have to trust that *it* knows, especially if the pregnancy ends up as a miscarriage or stillbirth.

Rabbi Herbert Weiner, who was a friend of ours for many years, told us a story about the *Angel of Forgetfulness*. He said that the Kabbalah identifies an angel who is present at the birth of every child. The angel touches the child on the upper lip, creating an indentation. This angel is the Angel of Forgetfulness. *The baby forgets what s/he has known before, and during, the gestational period and is born with a clean slate.* In my experience, there are many children now who must have been touched very lightly, because they DO remember and are aware of what transpired in utero and, sometimes, even prior to the pregnancy. I have written extensively about this phenomenon in my book *Born to Live*[178], so I will not go into greater detail about this here.

For many years, husbands were not allowed in or anywhere near the delivery room. Although my husband was a physician, our first four children were born without his presence. Therefore, I *chose* to have our last two children at home, so I could be in charge of who was present at their births. During the 1960's and early 1970's, many women wanted to have their babies at home, or at least have their husbands in the delivery room. Many husbands also wanted to be present. Since this was not acceptable in any of the Phoenix hospitals, we started a campaign in which my pregnant patients called the hospitals and asked if their husbands could be present in the delivery room. This campaign went on for a period of *twelve years* until, finally, Memorial Hospital in Phoenix began to allow husbands in the delivery room! Of course, birthing rooms are now very well-equipped and *whole families* can sometimes be present. I will never forget one birth in which a mother was having her seventh child, and all the other six children and her husband were present for the birth! As soon as the baby was born, they all spontaneously began to sing "Happy Birthday to You." This was such a happy time that the nurses and I were all in tears.

---

[178] McGarey, Gladys T., MD. Born to Live, 2008 (3rd ed.), Chapter 1 (p.1-9).

A friend created a school for autistic children, primarily because she has an autistic son and there were no educational facilities for children with this problem near where she lives. In her research she found that a great number of mothers of autistic children had had some very severe emotional and/or physical trauma when they were four months pregnant.[179] She remembered that at the time she was four months pregnant with *her* autistic child, her husband was having an affair with another woman. She subsequently had to live with her mother-in-law, who was very domineering and a difficult person to live with. While I realize we do not know what *all* the causes of autism are, this bit of retrospective research offers an interesting piece of information that should warrant further research.

During labor, a mother's thoughts and emotions are probably more in harmony with her total being—body, mind and spirit—than at almost any other time in her life. What she thinks, what she believes and what she has recognized about Life itself can be and is more readily able to be manipulated by and attuned to the movement of Life. To illustrate this idea, I want to share the story of a patient who suddenly began hemorrhaging after the birth of her child. The bleeding was very profuse, and I knew that we had to get an IV started immediately. But every time we put the needle in, her veins collapsed. I remembered that she had said she preferred no intervention whatsoever during the birth. She wanted to do it "naturally," without IV's or *anything* external in her body. It appeared to me that she was, in her *unconscious* state, creating a condition that resulted in us not being able to get an IV started. I also realized that if she had that kind of control over her body, she might be able to *stop* the bleeding. So, I said to her: "Linda, I want you to stop this bleeding, and I want you to stop it *right now.* You have control over your veins. You can control this bleeding. I want you to stop it *right now." Within two minutes, the bleeding stopped!*

Through the years, as I have worked with people who are being born and people who are dying, I have constantly been impressed

---

[179] Personal communication from the researcher to Dr. Gladys.

with the fact that *birth and death represent different sides of the same coin*. In both situations, our soul can choose the time, the place and the people it wants present for these transitions. I think it is important for us to understand that *any place where a person is born or dies becomes holy ground.*

When it is time for a baby to "awaken" or be born, s/he then moves through the vaginal canal and out into life. This movement through the birth passage is so like that of people who have had near-death experiences and report moving through a tunnel, that it poses an interesting parallel. To illustrate this point, Elisabeth Kübler-Ross (the physician who created the paradigm shift in how the medical world deals with death and dying) tells the following *birth* story. She said she had the feeling in utero that she was being squashed and hardly able to move, as if someone was sitting on her. Elisabeth was the first to be born of a triplet pregnancy, and I assume her other two siblings were perched on her shoulders most of the time, waiting to be born. During the birthing process, she recalled feeling pushed from above, as she moved through the birth canal. She also remembered how much she appreciated the love, tenderness and warmth of the physician's hands, as she and her two sisters were ushered into the world.

Another example comes to mind to illustrate this point. Once I was talking to a fifty-year-old Presbyterian minister. I had helped to birth him in Ohio and had seen him only occasionally in the years in between. He told me that all through his life he had had a feeling, a sensation, a "knowing" which he had been unable to identify until he was present at the birth of his first child. During *that* birth, he was able to recognize and identify those lifelong experiences as a memory from his own birth. He remembered a time when everything he had experienced in the womb up until a certain point began to shift. He felt like he was being squeezed and propelled forward in a way that he had no control over, and that it was something unavoidable. He felt like he was moving through the darkness towards the light. He remembered when the pressure began to ease off, and when he moved into the light. There was great jubilation and excitement in the world he came into. I remember his birth very clearly. His parents had three daughters and were truly jubilant when their *son* arrived.

Our souls seem to know that there comes a time when we let go of the old so we can move into the new. At birth, we move into the *physical* body, the vehicle through which we will find expression during this lifetime. In death, we let go of that vehicle and move into a dimension where our soul alone will be able to express itself. In both, we move through a dark tunnel, propelled by a force that we seem to have little conscious control over, almost as if we are squeezing out of the old to enter the new. In both situations, we are moving towards the light. *The people who are with us at the time of our birth and at the time of our death are the ones our soul has chosen to have there.* Time after time, we hear stories of a parent who could not die until a certain child was present (like what happened with Dr. Ann's mother). I have had the same experience in birthing babies.

Things may look new, feel new and sound new as we are born. On the other hand, when we die and let go of the five senses, we move into sensations of a *higher* vibration that probably also seems very new to us. As we make these transitions, we respond to those who are there to receive us. In either case, whether it is the arms of the mother and father on this plane or the presence of God on the other, it is possible to move into and behold the presence of Love. When we are born, we breathe in air and life; when we die, we exhale the air and breathe in Spirit. When we are born, the *umbilical cord* is cut, separating us from our mother. We become a separate individual. When we die, the *silver cord* is cut, separating us from Mother Earth, and we become an individual Spirit. Those who have had near-death or out-of-body experiences are aware of the presence of the silver cord. They realize that, if it were severed, they would not be able to return to their bodies. I find it interesting that, in most parts of the world, you need certificates for both birth and death!

Abortion represents a topic that is almost always explosive in nature, as the pros and cons of the subject come squarely into view. Personally, I have had difficulty trying to come to some sensible conclusions about this issue. *Spontaneous* abortion or miscarriage doesn't usually carry *the same* psychological impact or ethical tug-of-war that *elective* or *induced* abortion does. When it comes to a woman's *choice* to end her pregnancy, there are literally thousands of well-meaning men and women on *both* sides of the dividing line. For years I was torn between the two warring factions. In my mind, as the concept of the continuity of Life grew in its reality in *my* life, the pieces started to fall into place *for me. We have no beginning and no end as spiritual creatures.* Knowing this, I began to feel better about abortions that seemed to be necessary, as in the case of a woman having been raped and an unwanted pregnancy resulting. The idea of reincarnation helped. As I thought about how we *choose* our parents, how we *individually* view what lies ahead in our lives (no matter *what* it may be), and how life experiences serve our growth and understanding, I found myself beginning to understand the "pro-choice" point of view. However, I still had a problem with women who wanted an abortion because it was a convenient form of birth control, or because the pregnancy was embarrassing or threatened the stability of a marriage. These points of view did not make sense to me *personally*, as *I* had always been taught by my parents to follow through with whatever I started, *no matter what.* One day, though, a *new* awareness dawned in my consciousness, and the business of elective abortion became more understandable, *not* because I would choose to have an elective abortion myself, in my present level of awareness. Nevertheless, I can *now* see that it is frequently reasonable, understandable and the "right" thing for *some* women to do. (I will not get into the definition of "right" here.) This new awareness came to me from a story one of my patients told me some time ago,[180] and I share it here in hopes that it might help shed some light on this topic for others, as it did for me.

This mother had a four-year-old girl whom she would take out to lunch occasionally. During one such lunch, as they were talking about various things, the child began to shift from one subject to another. Suddenly, this child said: "The last time I was a little girl, I had a dif-

---

[180] McGarey, Gladys T., MD. Born to Live , 2008 (3rd ed.), p. 54-56.

ferent mommy!" She then began talking in a different language. Her mother quickly retrieved a pencil from her purse and copied down what her daughter had said, as nearly as she could understand it. Her daughter continued: "But that wasn't the last time. Last time, when I was this big [holding up her little index fingers about four inches apart] and in your tummy, Daddy wasn't ready to marry you yet, so I went away. But then, I came back." Her eyes lost that faraway look, and she began chatting again about four-year-old matters. The mother sat silent. *Only* her husband and her doctor knew that she had become pregnant about two years before she and her husband were ready to get married. When she was four months pregnant, she decided to have an abortion, because her husband-to-be was not yet ready to become a father. When the two of them did get married and both were ready to have their first child, the same entity evidently made its appearance. The little girl was saying, in effect: "I don't hold any resentment towards you for having had the abortion. I understood. I knew why it was done, and that's okay. So, here I am again. It was an experience. I learned from it, and you learned from it. So now, let's get on with the business of life *now*."

Perhaps the child did not have that kind of vocabulary. However, that was essentially what was being said by this four-year-old child in what she related to her mother. This mother's experience and the information from her four-year-old child *does* shine a new light on abortion, doesn't it? EVERY *experience is individual,* and not all abortions have this kind of circumstance surrounding them. In hearing this mother's experience, I could see how things were different than I first thought. *With birth and death, what we are dealing with is consciousness and the reality of consciousness.* Stories about *real* people help us to understand these aspects of Life. Since Love is the Great Healer, an abortion done for loving reasons is a healing, *living* process and *not* a killing action. (See my book *Born to Live* for a detailed discussion of this subject.[181])

---

[181] McGarey, Gladys T., MD. Born to Live , 2008 (3rd ed.), Chapters 6 and 7, p. 53-71.

Years ago, I had a wonderful couple as patients who were in their nineties. Esther had had a stroke and remained in the hospital for several weeks, unresponsive and connected to IV's. One day her daughter, a nurse who had worked in both hospice and home health, came to the hospital room and pulled up a chair next to her mother's bed. She said: "Ma, if you want to die, it's all right…you can go. You've had a good life, and if this is your time, it's all right for you to just leave. But, if you want to live, open your mouth and start eating *now*, because Dad and I will take care of you and take you home. But you *must* cooperate, and you *have to* open your mouth and start eating." Then the daughter sat back and waited. After about fifteen minutes, her mother's mouth began to move, and her daughter was able to give her some water. Gradually, her mother began to take sustenance and, within another week, they were able to take her home. Esther lived for another six months at home and then quietly died in her sleep. Harry lived to be 104. When he was 102, I asked him: "How are you doing, Harry?" He replied: "Just fine. My parents take care of me." I said: "What do you mean—parents?" He said: "Father Time, Mother Nature—they take care of me." He, too, died peacefully in his sleep.

My mother, who was eighty-nine years old and suffering from severe osteoporosis, was living in our home. On the Thursday before Easter, she was in the garden admiring the petunias, which were in a riot of bloom and color. When she returned to the house, she came in through the door and saw on the table the work that my father had been doing. He was putting together his book (see preface) and, on top of it all, sat a poster my oldest brother (John) had created when he was coming home from boarding school for the holidays. On the poster, in bold print, were the words: "Homeward Bound." Shortly after seeing that poster, my mother tripped and fell. My dad and I got her into an ambulance and admitted her into Scottsdale Memorial Hospital. My father stayed with her all night. The next day, around noontime, she said to him: "John, go get something to eat." He left to go down to the cafeteria for his lunch. After he left the room, she passed quietly. It was Good Friday. It was as if she could not leave with him being right there. They had enjoyed such a long, wonderful life together, and their lives were very much intertwined. It was hard for Dad to accept the fact that he was not there when she died. It was also hard for him to understand that she really could *not* go while he was there, because *his love was holding her on the earth plane.* When we went out to the cemetery for her interment, there was a gentle rain falling and a double rainbow across the sky. Two years after Mother died, my father married my brother's mother-in-law (Mother Daniels). This marriage became a little bit complicated, since it then made my brother and his wife brother and sister! Their son was coming home from Harvard for the wedding and told his professors he needed a leave because his grandparents were getting married! They said: "Don't you think it's about time?"

Dad and Mother Daniels had *both* enjoyed long and wonderful marriages, and now they were in a position where they could truly *play.* Neither one of them had ever taken the time just to play. They traveled for two years. Dad played shuffleboard and chess and put-tered with tools and woodwork. Mother Daniels quilted. They shared a wonderful life together. It was almost like their first marriages had been the cake, and this marriage was the icing. Then Dad got sick, and Mother Daniels knew that it was important for him to be in Phoe-nix with us, where my mother was buried. My husband and I thought maybe we would need a stretcher to get Dad off the plane. Not so! My strong, staunch, zealous, Presbyterian father was able to pull all his energy together and walk off the plane unassisted! We then had to put him in the hospital because he was so sick! He was there for two weeks and, one morning, Mother Daniels woke up and said: "I have to get to the hospital, and I have to get there *now.*" My sister-in-law took her to the hospital and, as Mother Daniels walked in the door, she realized that Dad was just about ready to make his transition. She stood by his bedside, held his hand and sang: "When the roll is called up yonder, I'll be there." His lips moved with hers as she sang. She continued singing: "God be with you 'til we meet again," as he made his transition. When I went to the hospital to bring her home, she said (through her tears): "Don't you know, there's jubilation on the other side?!" I knew that was true. I could just see my mother on the other side saying: "John, now it's time for you to come on over. You just come right on over, *now*." So, in *full* consciousness, Dad made his transition.

As strange as it may sound, humor can also play a role in these transitions. The following story of one of my patients illustrates this well. Lorraine Chase, PhD was the first psychologist to work with Art Linkletter on television. She and her husband were living in Scottsdale when she was diagnosed with lung cancer. Hospice was there to help her, and I made house calls. About two weeks before she died, I went to see her, and she said to me: "I know I'm medicated, and I know it probably would be considered a hallucination; but I looked up yesterday and saw that door." She pointed to a door that had two small panels at the top, with larger panels on the bottom, making a cross on the face of the door. She said: "I looked up and I saw Jesus on that cross, and I said to Him: 'Where have You been? I really, really have needed You.' He smiled and said: 'Right here.'" Then she said to Him again: "I really need help, and I wish that You would help me." Smiling, He reached down from the cross to touch her, with one arm and His back still on the cross. She said: "How did You do that?" He said with a smile: "Velcro." To me, the reality of this story is so important, because here we have a woman who is dying, and her sense of humor was so alive that she was able to joke with her God, who was also dying on the cross. What a powerfully wonderful way to make one's transition!

Another example of this kind of humor which occurred during the dying process was relayed to me after a lecture I gave. A woman came up to me and said that she was a hospice nurse. She had just experienced a situation in which an elderly mother was in a deep coma, surrounded by her grown children. One of the children said to her: "Mom, it's all right. Follow the light. Go to the light. It's all right." Suddenly, the dying woman opened her eyes, looked at her children, and said: "Will somebody please turn off that light? I'm not ready to go yet."

For some people, experiences in their bedrooms may not always remind them of pleasant memories. I have had patients who, for one reason or another, have been confined to their homes and unable to function in the outer world. For people like this, particularly if they have been active and creative in their lives previously, such a period of confinement can present a truly desperate time when their bedroom becomes a prison. One example of this is when a friend of mine who was an eighty-eight-year-old nurse died. She had been vitally active in her career, impacting the growth and evolution of holistic medicine. For years, she was known nationally for her ability to organize and present material. She was never presented with a project that she was unable to complete with great enthusiasm. When she developed lung cancer, however, letting *other* people take care of *her* became very difficult for her. She was physically and mentally active until about two weeks before she died. During this time, as her condition deteriorated, the one thing she kept repeating to her daughter was: "I guess I really need to learn to accept help." All her life she had been the one who helped *others*, and now her final lesson was to learn to *receive* help—a very difficult, yet profound, lesson. As she moved into a coma, periodically she would say to her daughter: **"I need to accept help." Sometimes this is the single, most important lesson that we must learn, even as physicians.**

People who are confined to their bedroom look for ways in which they can still be useful. As I listen to them, I realize that their physical problem can be a very difficult one. Along with this is their inability to see how they can contribute *anything at all* to our world. Because of this, I tell them the story of my brother Carl's experience in Bhutan.

Carl was a physician who had been active with the World Health Organization most of his professional life. He also created the Department of International Health at Johns Hopkins University. In 1962, he was invited by two physician friends to go to their country to see what could be done to improve the health of the Bhutanese people. During the month he was there, he was most impressed by the fact that every household in the country had a priest or monk visit them *every* day. He felt that if these priests and monks knew a little bit more about hygiene and nutrition, they would be able to help their people significantly. He talked to his physician friends about his idea and, although they felt it was a good idea, they told Carl that it would have to be first presented to the Great High Lama. Carl made the appointment with this holy man and described the journey to his abode like being in Shangri-La. They went through gardens and trellises and arches, higher and higher, until they came to a door. As they went through the door, they were told to prostrate themselves and move forward toward a dais on which there was a seated being of an undetermined age. Carl said this man's *body* was there, yet it felt as if *he* was not there. They stayed prone for a long period of time. Then, suddenly, the Great High Lama was back in his body and fully animated. He spoke to Carl and said he hoped he was having a good visit. Then he said: "You have a question." Carl presented the lama with his idea for the people. The lama said: "That's a good idea. I will have to take it into meditation." In an instant, he was "gone" again, although his body remained seated on the dais. Carl told us that, this time, the Lama was gone a *really* long time before he suddenly returned to his body again and said: "I have looked at the past. I have looked at the future, and I have taken this idea into consideration. *It is a very good idea, but the* timing *is wrong.* Right now, the forces of evil are mustering to enter the earth. If I took even one of my priests or monks away from his primary job, which is spiritual, and gave him a *physical* job, there would be an opening in the Universe that would allow the forces of evil to enter. I cannot do it right now." Carl said: "Thank you very much," and left. This was 1962, mind you, *before* Martin Luther King and John F. Kennedy were killed. About fifteen years later, they were able to do in Bhutan what Carl had suggested.

When I have told this story to people who had been homebound, they've responded with: "I can do as the lama suggests. I can pray for other people, and I know that's helpful." I say to them: "I would like you on my team, because I'm out in the world doing things all the time. However, to have someone like you who could keep me in your prayers, along with other people, would be a most helpful thing." One woman understood and said: "Particularly right now, with the world situation being what it is, I can see how my prayers could be very, very important in bringing about a healthier condition in our world, including world peace." Now, in light of current 2020 events, I think the prayers of people like this woman are needed more than ever.

One of the best things we can do for ourselves is to fall asleep with a prayer or a song of praise in our minds to allow our soul to move from the conscious into the unconscious, carrying with it a healing, *living* thought. When this happens, we are tapping into that Divine part of ourselves which truly allows rest to be recuperative and healing. Having done this one night, I awakened the next morning with this thought: *"May you have an uninterrupted day."* I then thought: "That's interesting." It became very clear to me that this thought was a very profound blessing. It allowed me to start my day with a sense of being blessed and in that space of attunement that is part of my soul connection with my Divine Self. If I have an *uninterrupted* day, it means that I can stay connected with the Physician Within me. Then, no matter what happens during the day, I will *still* be in that consciousness. I will not take into myself the difficulties and the trials that I *might* have to face that day, nor let them interrupt my day.

The bedroom is also the place where we symbolically need to take care of ourselves. No one else can lie down for us. No one else can sleep for us. There are certain things that we *must* do for ourselves. **When we neglect ourselves, we cannot *truly* help others**. In other words, **we need to take responsibility for *ourselves***. We need to treasure and respect this magnificent body in which we dwell. It is *truly* a temple of the Living God. In the words of my eldest daughter (Analea), it is "my body, my beloved."

Dreams also play an important part in our house of Living Medicine. It is in the bedroom where we most often encounter our *unconscious* self in dreams. We spend much of our life sleeping. As we sleep, our unconscious mind can help us with healing and rejuvenation. Also, through dreams, we can communicate with the deeper parts of ourselves. *Not addressing dreams in a book about Living Medicine would be like trying to talk about a life without sleep!* Dreams provide a fascinating way in which we can learn more about ourselves in an honest, safe way. I have found them to be tremendously helpful in working with patients. It helps me understand what they are going through. It also helps me to evolve therapeutic protocols and modalities that they can bring forth from *their* relationship with their Physician Within. The subject of dreams is far too complicated and vast to be dealt with adequately in this book. However, those of us in the health care field can use **the study of** our **dreams** and those of our patients **as a *profoundly* therapeutic and easily accessible tool to facilitate healing.** Even though patients *are the only ones who can* ultimately *interpret their dreams,* it is important to understand that they may need some help with this. If we as physicians learn this skill to help *ourselves* interpret our own dreams, we can then help our patients with *their* dream interpretations. Let me share a few examples to illustrate the importance of dreams.

A patient came to my office with a cold, and I suggested that she increase her intake of vitamin C. She called me the next morning to share a dream. In the dream, she was approaching her home carrying two bags of carrots. Just as she got to her door, a rotten lemon rolled off the roof of her house and landed in the bag of carrots. *What that dream told me was that she needed more vitamin A instead of additional vitamin C.* Another patient, who had struggled with depression all his life and had considered suicide several times, also shared a dream with me. He dreamt that he was standing on a rooftop with chimneys on top of it—*all kinds* of chimneys: thin ones, fat ones, ornate ones, plain ones, brick ones, stone ones. *Every chimney was different.* That rooftop with all those different chimneys extended as far as he could see into the horizon. Even though no two chimneys were alike, every so often there was one that was *incomplete.* Right before him stood one of the incomplete chimneys. In the dream, he knew that these chimneys represented people's lifetimes, and that this *specific,* incomplete chimney represented his current lifetime. He knew that if he did not complete this chimney in this lifetime, it would never, ever, ever be completed. *Because of that dream, he no longer considers shortening his life.* He still struggles with depression, yet he has never considered suicide again.

Some dreams can reflect how our destiny *can be changed without our even realizing it.* This happened to me, as the following example illustrates. One day I was shopping at the supermarket and, just as I pushed my cart through the door, it slammed shut on my right hand. I stood there for a while, because it was so painful. I was shaking my hand and watching a bruise grow on the back of it. I thought nothing more about it until a few days later. A pregnant patient of mine was in my office and asked: "What happened to you about two o'clock on Tuesday afternoon?" I replied: "Oh, nothing." Then she said: "I *know* something happened." I then remembered my experience in the grocery store and explained what happened to my hand. She said: "Well, that must have been it." Then she told me the following story. She was taking a nap and had a dream in which she saw me driving my car down the road and turning at the corner where the supermarket is located. Just as I turned the corner, a car sped through a red light, hit my car on the right side and hurt me very badly. She awakened, feeling very frightened for me, so began to pray for me for several minutes, until the feeling finally left. Her heart rate then slowed, and she was able to settle down. When she told me this, we realized that *her prayers probably intervened for me.* I believe that if I had *not* hurt my hand so badly that it required my attention for those few extra minutes in the store, I probably would have gotten immediately into my car. Had that happened, I would most likely have been at that intersection at the time when the car in her dream went through the red light. I truly believe that her prayers saved me from some severe trauma and should be viewed as what Dr. Ann calls a "Divine Delay."

The concept of the *collective unconscious* was originated by Carl Jung. It is defined as "the unconscious mind shared by all humanity."[182]

---

[182] Jung, Carl. The Archetypes and the Collective Unconscious, 1959.

The following story is a living example of this concept. Irene Hotten lived in Arvin, California with her husband (Mayo), who was an osteopathic physician (DO). One day, when she was helping her husband in his office, a woman who was an itinerant worker in the nearby fields came into the office. When she saw Irene, she said: "Oh my, *you* are the woman!" and then proceeded to tell Irene the following story. Six weeks prior to that time, this patient had been out in the field working and had fallen and fractured her ankle at dusk. She had no family or friends in the area yet managed to get herself into her room and up onto her bed. She was in a great deal of pain. Wondering what she should do, she began to pray for help. Suddenly, there was a woman standing at the foot of her bed. She looked at her clock and noticed it was eleven o'clock. This woman who had come into her room reached down, picked up her ankle, set the bones in the ankle and laid it back down on the bed. As the patient's pain eased, the woman left her bedside. Now, six weeks later, the patient was in Dr. Hotten's office for an X-ray to see if the bones had been properly aligned. They were, of course, completely aligned! The fascinating aspect of this story is that, every evening, when Irene did her meditation at just about eleven o'clock, she would pray for those who had no one to pray for them. In this case, *on an* actual *physical level, Irene was used to help this patient who was also praying for help at the* exact *same time.* Carl Jung called such experiences *synchronicity*, or "the coincidence in time of two or more causally unrelated events which have the same meaning."[183]

These last two stories were both connected with actual physical healings. Metaphorically, the bedroom is that place to which we can retire so that healing can take place. Both of the women in the last story were in states of consciousness similar to ones while in their bedrooms, which allowed them to remain in states of awareness where the body, mind and spirit are so in tune with each other that healing can happen on *any* level.

---

[183] Jung, CG. Synchronicity: An Acausal Connecting Principle, 2010.

Any time we move into a space of true *healing, it is like settling into our "bedroom consciousness."* The external cares are quieted, and sometimes even removed, as the "at-one-ment" (or attunement) takes place. This is how we allow healing to happen for ourselves and for those for whom we pray or to whom we minister. This bedroom consciousness can be tapped into at any time and from anywhere. **Healing energy is *always* available to us and to our patients, once we become conscious of this principle.** Knowing this, why would we as physicians ever *take* mind-altering medications, much less *prescribe* them to our patients (except in *extreme* circumstances)? It is the oath we all take as doctors: "**First, do no harm**," and I believe this oath applies equally to *ourselves* as well as our patients.

The above principle was never made clearer to me than when I went on a trip to China in 1966. I had been invited to tour this country as part of a team of thirty professional Arizona women participating in an exchange program with thirty professional women from China. For a month, we traveled around China visiting schools, factories, hospitals and other places of interest. At the end of the month, we went by train to Canton, after which we were to go to Hong Kong and then be on our way home. When we got off the train in Canton, the oldest woman in our group who was in her seventies, twisted her ankle so badly that she had a compound fracture. The Chinese people said that they would take her to the hospital. She said: "Absolutely not," so our team knew we had to do something to help her. In our group was a young woman who had just finished her orthopedic surgery training. She took one look at the woman's ankle, however, and walked away. She had absolutely no equipment with her and did not know how to deal with this fracture without at least having an X-ray machine. Since I was the only other physician on the team, it became my job to take care of the situation. The Chinese gave the woman some opium for the pain, which made her *quite* comfortable in the moment! However, I knew I *still* had to figure out what could be done for her ankle. Fortunately, the fracture was not bleeding a lot. I then asked two of the women in our group to give me their notebooks—each measuring about five by seven inches, and a couple of their scarves. With a great deal of prayer and trepidation, I put both of my hands around her ankle and very gently guided the bones back into their correct positions. Not being able to see how much damage I had to deal with, *I had to trust the patient's body responses* in my efforts to reposition the fractured bones.

Since we were on a tight time schedule, the rest of the group had to go across the railroad bridge from Canton to Hong Kong, leaving me with the Chinese team and the patient. Before we had left Phoenix, I had talked to Dr. Pearl Chang, who was Chinese and someone I had worked with previously in Phoenix. Dr. Chang had a brother who was the head of a radiation department in Hong Kong. She had given me his phone number when we had met, in case our team might need some help while we were in China. So I called Dr. Chang's brother and told him the situation. He said he would send an ambulance to meet us on the other side of the bridge. This meant I had to get the patient (by stretcher) to the middle of the bridge, so that the people from the ambulance could transfer her to it and get her to Hong Kong. Dr. Chang's brother said that it would take about an hour for the ambulance to get there, so I was left to care for this patient while we waited. Fortunately, the patient was still *quite* comfortable from her opium dose and feeling no pain! I, on the other hand, was praying a lot and feeling very uncertain about what was really happening to her ankle, since she was feeling no pain at all. I wondered if I had severed her nerves in my attempt to reset her bones and worried that her level of comfort might be due to that or something other than the opiate. We waited the hour and, sure enough, the ambulance arrived at the other end of the bridge. This bridge ran over the Shenzhen (also called Sham Chun) River that separates the natural border of Hong Kong from Mainland China.[184] In reality, this bridge was only a "motorable road" that was hurriedly built to connect the railway systems of the two countries in order for military supplies to be transported into

---

[184] www.en.m.wikipedia.org>Sham_Chun_River.

China from Hong Kong after the Japanese attack in 1937.[185] So, the train tracks were not really a bridge, they were just the tracks that went over this deep waterway, and the water was *quite* a ways down!

It was a *tremendous challenge* for me to get the patient to the middle of the bridge so that she could be transferred from the stretcher to the ambulance. It meant that the *Chinese* men had to carry her on the stretcher to the transfer point in the middle of the bridge. It also meant that *I* was the one left to carry our luggage! This luggage consisted of all the large string bags that the patient and I had accumulated during the month, which contained our gifts for family and friends. To accomplish this task, I hung these large bags on the ends of a pole that I had to carry across my shoulders, while I carried our suitcases and our purses by hand. I had to walk in this manner across the train tracks, taking one slow step at a time to keep my balance, having a clear view of the water *far* below me the entire time. Fortunately, I am not afraid of heights, so we both made the trip across the bridge successfully.

When we got to Hong Kong, Dr. Chang's brother met the ambulance, and we got the patient into the X-ray room. After the X-ray was done, to my delight and amazement the film showed that there were five segments of bone, *all properly aligned* in the patient's ankle! All Dr. Chang's brother had to do then was to order a good cast to put on her leg and ankle. She then stayed in Hong Kong for another six weeks before she flew home.

I did not see the patient again until a couple of years later, when we ran into each other in downtown Scottsdale quite by accident. I asked her how she was feeling since our trip to China. She then told me the following story. When she came home after her extra six weeks in Hong Kong, she said she was feeling fine and was able to walk around very well without any pain. *She then went to see her orthopedic doctor, who had trouble believing that her ankle had been set properly following her compound fracture.* He then X-rayed her ankle from which he interpreted that there was some misalignment

---

[185] Chan, Ming K. and John D. Young. Precarious Balance: Hong Kong Between China and Britain, 1942-1992. (reprinted in 2015).

still present in her ankle. He then told her she needed surgery (an open reduction) to correct this misalignment. According to the patient, *after he did that surgical procedure, she has never been free of pain in that ankle.* In my mind, had the patient's orthopedic surgeon been able to tap into *his own* Physician Within from a "bedroom consciousness" state, he might *not* have felt the need to schedule this surgical procedure for the patient at the six-week mark in her healing process. He *might* have considered waiting for the injury to *fully* heal and *then* re-evaluate her ankle at *that* time, before deciding that she needed that surgery.

The bedroom can also be the literal place where the Physician Within can contact the Physician Without in a very profound and comfortable way. When I was making house calls, some of the most tender moments I *ever* had with patients occurred at their bedside in their home. *This principle also holds true* when we are at the bedside of patients in the hospital. This can likewise happen when patients come into our office and we share that still, quiet place symbolized by the *consciousness* of the bedroom.

In summary, the bedroom in our house of Living Medicine can become a place in our lives *where our unconscious and our conscious meet.* It is also where transitions happen. In this state, where our awareness of the connection between body, mind and spirit can become *very* real, we move in and out of our *conscious* reality. Said in a slightly more humorous way, the bedroom can *literally* become the room in our Living Medicine dwelling place where we can *consciously* experience our lives "from lust to dust."

7

The Playroom

The house of Living Medicine would be incomplete without a play-room! One of the most important aspects of maintaining a healthy life is *balance*. **Balance between work and play is *pivotal* to the proper movement of Life energy for *both* physicians and patients.** By play I mean that which brings joy and laughter, as well as relaxation and being physically involved with the *living* energy of Spirit that enlivens us all. Play can involve others or can be an individual and personal activity. Setting aside a place for this activity not only validates it, it affirms on a material level that this room is as important as any other room in the house.

When the children of Israel received the Ten Commandments, one of them was: "Remember the Sabbath Day to keep it holy. Six days shalt thou labor and do all thy work, but the seventh day is the Sabbath of the Lord thy God. In it, thou shalt not do any work" (Exodus 20:8-11). The Sabbath symbolizes the importance of taking time away from our "work." In the context of the Ten Commandments, we should dedicate one out of seven days to the *enjoyment* of life and the movement of the Spirit within us. Perhaps, in today's world, we cannot find a *whole* day every week to which we can dedicate this kind of time. However, we certainly can understand *the importance of taking time* each *day to allow our body, mind and spirit to just enjoy each other.*

We have become very aware that *exercise* **is important for the proper functioning of the body**. Exercise in any form that does not *over*extend our abilities is effective and essential to our well-being. Based on Dr. Ann's personal experience and research,[186] however, the *important distinction* lies in the definition of what exercise *really* is. She was challenged to look at this distinction by one of her patients, a Feldenkrais practitioner, who told her he thought he knew what exercise was until he did some serious research on this topic. Dr. Ann was particularly interested in this conversation after receiving some DNA test[187] results that told her what kind of exercise was *ideal* for her genetic profile; and it *wasn't* what she had been doing all her life! Intrigued and determined to figure this out, she contacted a personal trainer who *does* understand this distinction *and* who also does the *kind* of exercise that Dr. Ann's test results had *specifically* recommended for her. Consequently, she *exercises* once a week and participates in *recreational activities* the rest of the time! She found this distinction to be a *huge* relief, knowing that she was *now* doing what her body *needed* and would respond *best* to for exercise instead of what she had always thought she *should* do and not always enjoying. This distinction was such a revelation to her *personally*—and, as it turned out, to *many* of her patients—that she now teaches the following distinctions to her patients. As a result, many of her patients who had stopped exercising because they didn't "enjoy" it are now willing to include exercise into their lives once again. To help her patients make this decision, she gives them a handout containing the following information.[188]

"In a nutshell: **EXERCISE** *is a process* *whereby the body performs work of a* **de-manding** *nature,* **[where] muscular loading**

---

[186] McGuff, Doug, MD and John Little. Body by Science: A Research Based Program for Strength Training, Body Building and Complete Fitness in 12 Minutes a Week, 2009.

[187] DNA Testing, jfreiberg@rx@live.com (99.9 % accurate).

[188] Hutchens, Ken. "Exercise vs. Recreation.pdf," Super Slow®: The Ultimate Exercise Protocol, 1992.

must render momentary muscular failure within one to three minutes." *In addition,* exercise "is either piecemeal or nonexistent [if it doesn't produce *continuous* improvement in the] *six factors of physical fitness:* muscular size, strength and endurance; bone strength; cardiovascular efficiency; enhanced flexibility; and a contribution to body leanness. **RECRE-ATION**, on the other hand, is a different matter altogether. It **is fun, [includes] pastime activities, [is] a diversion from daily routine...** and *very* **important to our mental health.**"

Five Distinctions Between
Exercise and Recreation

EXERCISE	RECREATION
Logical	Instinctive
Universal	Personal
General	Specific
Physical	Mental
Not fun	Fun

"**Do not try to make exercise enjoyable. Do not try to make recreation exercise.** If you confuse and mix exercise and recreation, you grossly compromise any forthcoming *physical* benefits of the exercise; you destroy a large degree of the fun that recreation can bestow; and you make both more dangerous than they need be. *Accept both for what they are.* If you can place exercise and recreation in their *proper* perspective, the quality of your life will markedly improve."

Play enriches our lives. Based upon the above information, I believe that we need to find the type of play (recreation) that we, as individuals, *truly* enjoy. When we do this, it becomes a *healing* activity as well as fun. The more we understand the differences between exercise and recreation/play and accept them, the more we can participate in *both* wholeheartedly. In so doing, our body, mind *and* spirit can *truly* benefit from *both* of these activities as healing experiences.

Our form of play may be quilting, knitting, gardening, listening to music, dancing, playing family games or even watching television. We have untold numbers of ways in which we can be entertained. *There is nothing wrong with* any *form of play as long as it isn't our* only *form of play.* If it requires something from the *outside* to stimulate our Life Force, however, we become dependent on *outer* stimulation to keep us engaged in life.

For some people, a form of play has manifested in re-creating their bodies. For many years, I have seen an increase in the amount of body mutilation that people are inflicting upon themselves—piercings, tattoos and even excessive plastic surgery. *I have wondered what the people involved in these activities are looking for and what they think they are missing.* I approach this discussion *not* from the place of judgement or condemnation. Rather, my interest lies in trying to understand what that particular person wants to express. *For many years now we have given ourselves so many ways to distract ourselves from real connection —to ourselves, to others and to the Divine.* We have done this through video games, movies and all types of sensory stimuli, including all forms of social media. It seems to me that these distractions have, in many cases, resulted in a situation of sensory overload, so that we cannot really *feel* without having to go beyond the "normal" sensory input. I wonder if those who pierce their tongues are trying to say something that they want to say yet cannot express adequately. Or if those who have *multiple* piercings in their ears are trying to hear something that goes beyond what they have been listening to. In wondering about this relatively recent phenomenon, I came across an article by Larry Dossey, MD.[189] I believe his article of-

---

[189] Dossey, Larry, MD. "Living Dangerously, Risk-Taking and Health," Alternative Therapy, Nov-Dec 2003.

fers a thought-provoking and important piece of information to help us understand what may be happening in this realm. He writes: "The eternal job of the writer is to comfort the afflicted and afflict the comfortable." He goes on to describe our human need for stretching beyond our "comfort zone" and puts it into the context of our basic innate nature, which is to allow risk in our lives. In his article, Dossey says (italics are mine) : *"The grail quest is a symbolic journey,* toward a psychological awakening and enlightenment. It champions and celebrates risk. It teaches us that a quest without it is not genuine but is an exercise in self-indulgence." *I wonder if the desire to "recreate" our bodies could be the result of the loss of such a quest.*

We, as parents, naturally want to remove danger from our children's lives, and this is commendable. However, how are our children going to learn to ride a bicycle if we do not put them on it and let them fall? How can we possibly create a risk-free world without damaging that inner urge that needs to be expressed? Dossey goes on to say: "We have created diagnostic categories for rambunctious, risk-loving boys and have taken to rationalizing boyish behavior out of existence. We prefer, instead, perfectly behaved, undisruptive kids who grow up to be mellow, smoothed-out adults."

Our desire to eliminate risk in our lives is an attempt to eliminate fear. In the attempt to take fear away, we create greater and greater fears. We compound our fears and do not transform them. The classic statement: "Why worry when you can pray?"[190] is lost in a world of worries and fears that are constantly with us. "As politicians have learned, we are easy to scare, but impossible to un-scare," Dossey says. I believe that the only way to deal with worry and fear is *not* to try and eliminate them. A better way for us to deal with worry and fear is to *face* them, *deal* with them and *move through* them instead of avoiding them. Every day that I work with patients I am constantly humbled by the magnificence of the human spirit as they walk through their "valley," whether it be cancer, a broken home or death itself.

---

[190] Peale, Norman Vincent. Why Worry When You Can Pray?, 1961.

In medicine, we have put up so many barriers and walls in the process of trying to avoid litigation that *most physicians live in a constant state of fear, and their practice of medicine is directed by trying to avoid all risk*. Dossey also addresses this condition in his article [bold is mine].

> *Many of us physicians remember when patients and physicians felt they were on the **same** side, and we wonder if things can ever be that way again. For that to happen, we shall need, I believe, to give up the fantasy that healthcare can be **both** effective **and** error-free and that risk can always be assigned to specific individuals. In healthcare, risk and safety are like the opposite poles of the magnet, without which the magnet could not exist. Perhaps that's why nature seems to laugh at our attempts to eliminate risks completely. **Risk is a paradox**, which has been defined as truth standing upside down to attract attention. This paradox is our birthright and a reminder that our obsession with creating a risk-free existence from the nursery to the crematory is folly.*

I am *not* saying we should not be cautious and not take precautions. Risk is the aspect of awareness that we all crave and need, and which pulls us past the safety zone of comfort and moves us into the reality of Life itself. It allows us to move into a life that enhances play and the joy of life.

One of the problems we are experiencing in life is *addictions*, whether it is to drugs, alcohol or social media. I have heard about video games that are so "real" that people get completely caught up. It then becomes hard for them to participate in real-life relationships. *The personal identity they create in their game (their avatar) is one that they like and have power over, which then makes them feel like they have power over others.* **Dreaming and daydreaming offer ways in which** our creative energy flows and grows. **However, when it becomes difficult getting *out* of the fantasy world and returning to the functional world, it becomes pathological.** *We do not want creative children disrupting the classrooms, so we medicate them to keep them in line.* We overwork our teachers, so they do not have the time or patience to help direct *their own* creative energy. We also overcrowd the classrooms. The great minds of our youth are also sometimes either addicted to something or medicated. As a result, they have trouble really allowing themselves to get *truly* zealous about *any* cause.

Allowing children to get hot, sweaty and dirty so they can experience how great a shower feels is important. Let them participate in *other people's* loss and hunger, so they can know how blessed *they* are. Let them feel *their own* pain and loss, and then help them face and grow through *their* experiences. Sometimes medication *may* be needed, however, it should not be the *first* thing that we use. Let children take responsibility for *their own* healing, yet be available when they need us. We cannot digest our children's life experiences *for* them, that is something they must do *for themselves*.

As we give ourselves room in this house of Living Medicine for play, it is important to accept and realize the importance of *unstructured* play—taking time just to BE and enjoy the essence of whatever IS. Sometimes we get so caught up with the *busyness* of our lives that we lose the spontaneity of unstructured or spontaneous play. For example, as an eight-year-old boy my son (Bob) would literally spend *hours* playing with ants in the backyard of our home. Once he found an anthill and was so fascinated with the ants' activity that he decided he was going to help them build a community. He made pathways and bridges, sprinkling a little bit of food along the way, watching them follow the paths he had created. For me, just watching *him* play with those ants was an act of joyful relaxation!

There should always be room for play in our house of Living Medicine, which means *time to do nothing*, at least nothing considered constructive, whatever that "nothing" might be for each person. We criticize our children in school for daydreaming, and yet some of the most important concepts and life-changing experiences have resulted from it. Einstein was a perfect example of this.[191] *Daydreaming is such a natural process for us that we tend to discredit and downplay it.* When we create school buildings that have no windows for the children to look outside, we restrict their ability to daydream. In doing this, we really deprive them of the growth of their Spirit by not allowing them to stretch and grow as they would if allowed to daydream.

When I practiced medicine in Wellsville, Ohio in the early 1950's, my brother and his family lived about thirty-five miles away in Pennsylvania. One day, I went to visit them with my four children, including my son (Carl) who was five years old at the time. I had three sons and a daughter, and my brother had three daughters. When we got back from the visit, Carl was at his toy box, pulling his toys out and arranging them. I asked him what he was doing. His answer was: "Poor Uncle John. His kids don't have any toys at all. I'm finding the toys we can give to them." Now, of course this was because all he saw at Uncle John's house were *girls'* toys, and he was feeling very sorry for his girl cousins who just did not have trucks or balls or sticks or boy stuff. My five-year-old son was reaching out to his girl cousins in a loving, tender way and, for this, I was grateful. However, I had to explain to him that his *girl* cousins really were not into trucks and that, maybe, there were some *other* things we could think about giving them rather than those boys' toys that were so precious to him.

I have thought about this story as a metaphor for a number of things that have happened in my own life. How often have I projected my own needs and desires on other people when *their* needs and desires may have been completely different? How often did I feel sorry for somebody and want to give them something from my compassionate heart that would have been important and helpful to *me*, though might have been useless and maybe not at all appropriate for *them*? We project our own wishes and emotions and thoughts on other people because we feel they need them, or we feel *they* are lacking. In reality, though, *they* have not felt the lack *or* the need and have not asked for our opinion or

---

[191] http:m.natgeotv.com/int/genius/videos.

even our pity. *When we use our own desires to help someone else and do not listen to what they are saying, do not pay any attention to what their needs are or even try to understand where they are coming from, we frequently create more trouble than help.* A perfect example of this is what gets donated during disasters: "approximately sixty percent of items donated after a disaster *can't be used*"[192,193] to help those in need.

The idea that *we* know what is best for other people because it would be best for *us* was brought forcefully to my attention in the early 1950's when I lived and practiced in Wellsville, Ohio. The business-women in Wellsville and East Liverpool had formed an organization called the Quota Club, which had as its mission doing things in our hometowns that would be helpful for the people. We took on projects that were geared towards making the city a better place to live. One of these projects included the health care and well-being of several old men, who were almost or completely blind and lived in shacks on the banks of the Ohio River. Out of the kindness of our hearts, we wanted to help these men improve their living conditions. We rented a house with enough rooms to accommodate *everyone*, hired a housekeeper, furnished the house with bedding and dishes and anything else we felt was necessary to make them comfortable. We then went down and talked to the men. We offered them this place to live, saying that *we* would take care of their housing, since we felt they would do better in a different situation. We even took them to the house and showed them around. They were *not* enthusiastic and did *not* move into the house. We waited a few days and then felt that the reason they had not accepted our offer was because they did not know how great it would be to have clean sheets and a nice place to live. So we went and bodily moved them into the house. They stayed there almost two weeks, and then *every one of them* went back to their shacks by the riverside! We could not believe it. We were absolutely astonished that

---

[192] Fessler, Pam. "Thanks, But No Thanks: When Post-Disaster Donations Overwhelm" (www.npr.org>2013/01/09>thanks-but-no>thanks).

[193] Gruberg, Shabab. (www.good360.org>impact-stories>the-second>disaster>of>im practical>donations – Sept 14, 2020).

the opportunity we had given them was *totally* rejected and that they could go back to the conditions that were, in *our* minds, unhealthy.

I have never forgotten this experience. It pointed out to me that there was a certain arrogance in my attitude. I had assumed that *I* knew what these men wanted and needed in *their* life situation, instead of simply asking them what *they* wanted and needed. **In helping people with their healing, we need to know** *their* **wishes and needs.** Someone who clearly understood this principle and did what our Quota Club failed to do was Pastor Mack McCarter. He is the founder and coordinator of Community Renewal International (CRI) in Shreveport, Louisiana.[194] After being a pastor in Texas for many years, he returned to his hometown of Shreveport in 1991 following the news and outcome of the 1988 race riot there. The CRI website describes: "He found many of its once vital and thriving neighborhoods...in decline." The badly-hurting community was "dealing with gangs, drugs, violence, crumbling homes ['shotgun rowhouses'] and people living in isolation. Believing the situation could be healed, he founded CRI in 1994 with one goal in mind: to rebuild his hometown by uniting individuals, churches, businesses and civic groups through resurrecting the foundation of relationships in neighborhoods." He accomplished this goal by "tapping into two inherent human needs —to love and be loved—[to] make people feel safe, confident and optimistic." Because of CRI, crime has dropped in some of Shreveport's neighborhoods by as much as fifty-two percent. "One of the pillars of our work is to *bring folks together based on what they share in common, not how different they are.* What we [all] share in common is [the] God-given capacity to care for one another and be cared for." Neighborhoods are united and recognized for their efforts by placing "We Care" signs in their yards and bumper stickers on their cars. His team of volunteers exceeds fifty thousand and his CRI model has now spread to other U.S. cities and across the globe.[195] In light of recent events in 2020, we think this model holds real promise to help heal systemic racism once and for all.

---

[194] www.CommunityRenewal.us>us>Mack-McCarter and ...>project.

[195] www.crux.com>2019/10>catholic-extension-honors-Louisiana-faith-leader-for-uniting-communities.

I think we must be mindful of this principle also as a nation. We must be careful not to make the types of assumptions our Quota Club made in our dealings with other countries. Instead of trying to force upon them *our* idea of democracy, perhaps we should be asking what it is *they* need, as Mack McCarter did. The reason Future Generations, an organization started by my brother (Carl) and his son (Dan), has been so effective around the world is because they identify what *the people themselves* want, not what *they* think the people should have. I wonder how often we force our own precious ideologies and philosophies onto people for whom they are either useless or inappropriate?

We live in a world where taking time to slow down or just relax is sometimes very difficult. The following story is one that I heard as a child, which still has great meaning to me to this day. It seems that one of my father's friends, a fellow missionary, was trekking back into the jungle with *coolies* (people whose jobs it is to do whatever work needs to be done) carrying his equipment. After they had traveled for three days, he was all set and ready to go the morning of the fourth day. However, the coolies remained sitting. He told them that they needed to move on, that they had a schedule to meet and so on. The coolies just sat there. He continued to try to persuade them. He finally told the head man that he *really* needed to get them to continue with the trek. At this point, the head man said: "Sahib, these men have left their souls behind for three days, and they're waiting for them to catch up. They will not move until their souls have caught up." I have often wondered whether that idea can explain jet lag! I also wonder if the inability to understand ourselves and our fellow human beings has a great deal to do with the *pace* at which we live our lives. Perhaps if we slowed down, *our* souls would have a chance to catch up with *us!* Could it be that this is part of what this 2020 coronavirus pandemic is all about?

I think that we *all* should have a rocking chair where we simply sit and rock, or a swing on which we can swing back and forth. This rhythmic motion is very beneficial to our bodies physically. These movements promote circulation and help us work into our lives a rhythm that is part of the healing process. *The gentle movement of the rocking chair or the swing serves to activate the lymphatic sys-tem.* President John F. Kennedy found great relief from his back pain using his rocking chair.[196] I think one of the reasons the elderly enjoy the rocking chair is because it allows a movement that is pleasant and soothing, while enhancing the circulatory and lymphatic systems. Babies respond to rocking from the moment they are born. This is understandable since, *in utero,* whenever a mother walks or moves, the baby feels a movement like that of being rocked.

The playroom can provide a place where beauty in *any* form can be appreciated. *Beauty is different for each one of us.* As we accept our *own* individuality, we become aware of ourselves and our own *inner* attunement. *To set aside a time and place in our busy lives where we really do appreciate the beauty around us is essential to the growth of our* spiritual *nature.* There is also growing evidence docu-menting the importance of the *physical environment* in the healing process.[197,198,199] That is why our planned *Village for Living Medicine*—a groundbreaking, state-of-the-art healing campus with programs to be based upon the philosophical framework of Living Medicine —will be sensitive to and enhance the beauty of the land upon which it will be erected. Its building designs, construction and landscaping will of-fer a *living* environment that promotes healing through beauty, art, music, color, light and other elements that inspire hope and feed the Spirit. The following story identifies how *each* of us can access these aspects in *our own* lives that allow us to grow and heal.

I had a friend who came into my office and relayed a dream, which she said she knew was very, very important and *insisted* that I had to tell other people about it. In the dream, she saw a three-sided rectan-gle with the words "love, stress, pain and beauty" displayed as shown

---

[196] Hamilton, E.L. "Youthful President JFK relied on old-fashioned rocking chairs to relieve his back pain," www.thevintagenews.com>2018/05/09.

[197] Huisman, E.R.C.M. et.al. (2012). Healing environment: A review of the impact of physical environmental factors on users. Building and Environment. 58.70-80. 10.1016/j.buildenv.2012.06.016.

[198] https://doi.org/10.1080/09613218.2017.1411130.

[199] https://www.ncbi.nlm.nih.gov>pmc4424933.

in the diagram below. When she told me this dream, I really did not know what to do with it.

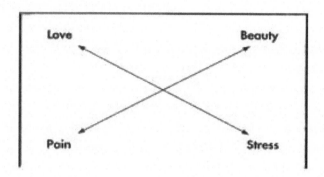

The following week I went to the symphony with this same friend. She was having a great deal of back pain at the time. Sitting through the first two compositions made the pain in her back *very* uncomfortable. The third composition (by Schubert), however, affected her so deeply that ALL *the pain in her back went away by the end of the performance of that piece, and she remained pain-free for some twelve hours afterwards.* It was apparent that beauty and pain were somehow connected in her body. The beauty of the music, the depth at which she experienced its vibration in her body, as well as that specific music itself, helped her transcend her pain for the next twelve hours. Two weeks later, it was Mozart's music that moved her out of her pain. The fact that the rectangle was open at the bottom told me that this illustration represented a principle that could be applied to anyone. It also told me that it was *not* just an isolated, individual experience. It seemed that, **if people can move into whatever their appreciation of beauty is, it will help them transcend their pain.** This principle has been validated by the work of the Therapeutic Harp Foundation in Phoenix, Arizona; a group of harpists who play their instruments for terminally and chronically ill patients. Because of their music, patients have been able to cut back on their use of pain medications, particularly OxyContin.[200] During 2020, they are partnering with the largest health care network in the

---

[200] www.theharpfoundation.org.

U.S. to conduct additional research. Even though I haven't addressed the love/stress connection in this example, the research in this area of my friend's dream diagram is well-documented. The groundbreaking research of Dr. Hans Selye[201] (1907-1982) showing **stress** to be **THE underlying cause of almost all chronic illness** has stood the test of time and remains as relevant today as ever.

Another paradigm from which to view the origin of illness and principles of healing is the Edgar Cayce readings on health and healing.[202,203] One of these fundamental principles is *self-responsibility*.[204] This means that **we are EACH *individually responsible* for the health of *every* cell of our body.** Said another way: *it is the consciousness of the ME that takes care of each cell.*

Thus, the nourishment that we give ourselves on *all* levels—body, mind and spirit—is up to *each one* of us. Cayce also said: "all healing, mental or material, is attuning *each atom* of the body [and] *each reflex* of the brain forces, to the awareness of the Divine that lies within each atom [and] each cell of the body.[205] To that end, we are *individually* responsible for providing the *best quality* of nutrients to our cells that we can *and* for removing waste from them as efficiently as possible. One of the benefits of using a castor oil pack is that it gives us the *opportunity* to slow down and take time out to allow our physical body to absorb the castor oil. Doing this helps the cells of our *whole* body (*including the nervous system*) rid itself of toxins via the lymphatic system. I will never forget a young boy named Timmy who brought this important principle to my attention.

The first time Timmy came into my office, I heard him before I saw him! He was *not* crying or screaming…he was just tearing the room apart! When I stepped into the examining room, I saw a young mother who was *totally* frustrated by her adorable five-year-old child. We *were*

---

[201] https://ncbi.nlm.nih.gov>pmc5915631.

[202] www.edgarcayce.org>holistic>health>database.

[203] www.edgarcayce.org>circulating>file>principles>of>healing.

[204] Thurston, Mark, PhD. "Introduction to the Cayce Readings on Health and Healing," www.EdgarCayce'sA.R.E.>The>Readings>Health>and>Wellness>Holistic>Health>Database>Health>and>Healing:Introduction.

[205] www.edgarcayce.org. Reading 3364.2.

able to talk over the uproar about his health, which was basically excellent, except for chronic constipation and frequent bouts of sore throats and earaches that required antibiotics. I tried to get a history of his diet and found that he consumed a great deal of sugar, milk and foods with preservatives. I suggested changes in his diet, which his mother was open to doing. When he came into the office a month later, his *activity* was just as wild, though he had not experienced a sore throat and had had a little less trouble with his ears during that month. However, *his constipation remained severe.* I suggested to his mother that she start using a castor oil pack on his abdomen. Since he had trouble holding still, we decided to put the pack on from four to five in the afternoon while he watched a local television program for children. *About a month later, when he came into the office again, I did not even know he was there!* When I went into the examining room, Timmy was quietly turning pages in a book. I was really delighted and amazed. His mother said that *the castor oil packs had made all the difference.* She continued to use them as Timmy started school. She discontinued them in the summertime, though periodically he would come running in and say: "Mama, I need the pack! I need the pack!" Throughout his school years, there would be times when he would come home and tell his mother he "needed the pack." It seems that he could feel when the tension began to build up in his system. He knew he would not be able to control it and that the castor oil pack would help. I have since seen him in my office as a grown man with children of his own, perfectly capable of continuing his life and activities and raising a healthy family.

In our society, there are many children who are on medications because of *hyperactivity.* These children learn that they can control their feelings and behavior with the use of pills. Sadly, many of them continue using other prescription drugs in their later years. How much better it would be if we could **find ways to *effectively* treat the PROBLEM, whatever it is, instead of just suppressing the *symptoms* of the problem with prescription medications**.

In the playroom, we can also reconnect with concepts that result from nursery rhymes and fairytales. The field of *conventional* medicine could very easily be portrayed in the nursery rhyme: "There was an old woman who lived in a shoe. She had so many children, she didn't know what to do. She gave them some milk without any bread and whipped them all soundly and put them to bed." The old woman lives in one shoe. She cannot walk, and she cannot move or go anywhere with just *one* shoe. *She needs to find another shoe before she can walk.* Conventional medicine has moved into the consciousness of being confined to one shoe in working with issues that are really *life* issues yet are dealt with only as *health* issues. The old woman, representing *conventional* medicine, is working very hard to keep all the concepts within controlled boundaries. *No wonder conventional physicians feel so boxed in!* Conventional medicine tries to understand and deal with all the *diseases* that humankind has *ever* seen. There are, however, *so many* children's diseases that it is impossible to control them. The old woman just does *not* know what to do. She is tired, angry and frustrated, just like many physicians feel today. **Conventional medicine, in the way it is being practiced currently, faces that same dilemma: it just "[does not] know what to do,"** including during this 2020 COVID-19 pandemic. The old woman gives the children "some milk without any bread and whipped them all soundly and put them to bed." In *conventional* medicine, we treat the diseases the same way: administering therapies that control *symptoms*. It does *not* deal with the *underlying cause(s)* of those symptoms. We need more sustenance or deeper healing. We need some aspect of Spirit or "Bread of Life." Because *diseases* do not act the way we would like them to, we "[whip] them all soundly and put them to bed." We try to *control the disease* by primarily addressing the *symptoms*, not really allowing healing an opportunity to happen. We "whip" the symptoms into submission and then move on to the *next* patient, which is the description of "managed care" in a nutshell! Attempting to deal with the underlying *causes* of the patient's symptoms then becomes very difficult. *When we are only allowed enough time to deal with the* symptoms *of diseases in this currently very broken health "care" system known as "managed care,"* true *healing becomes* almost *impossible.*

Our *health* care system is now mostly a system of "disease" care. **Our challenge as physicians then becomes a *never-ending process* of trying to quiet the *symptoms.* Not addressing the *underlying cause* of those symptoms prevents the opportunity for *true* heal-ing to occur.** As physicians, we need to find the "other shoe," which *I* believe is Living Medicine, and *it is within arm's reach.* Like the old woman in the nursery rhyme, we just need to *look* for it. I wrote about this principle in an article[206] entitled "Focusing on Health, Not the Dis-ease," and is excerpted below:

> *Andrew Taylor Still, the founder of osteopathy said: "To find health should be the object of the doctor. Anyone can find disease." For many years, I have had the privilege of working with a lady who is a dancer and a healer. She came to my office for a check-up. She is a wonder-ful person who, for many years has worked with concepts from the Edgar Cayce material and has been dealing with a physical problem called **polycythemia rubra vera.** When this diagnosis was first made, it sounded to her like she was being given a death sentence. She was told that it was a terminal illness and was something that would have to be treated for the rest of her life. This prognosis was ac-companied by the only path of conventional medicine treatment open to her, which was medication and regular phlebotomies (blood-letting). I saw her shortly after she received this news. She believed that the Physician Within her knew a great deal about her body and would have something to add to her ther-*

---

[206] McGarey, Gladys Taylor, MD. "Focusing on Health, Not the Disease," Venture Inward: The Magazine of the A.R.E. and the Edgar Cayce Foundation, April 2013.

*apy. At the time, she was having severe mus-
cular spasms, joint pain, debilitating fatigue
and drenching sweats. As an artist, she called
on her ability to visualize and began to picture
her red cells reproducing themselves in their
own natural way and time, and her body rid-
ding itself of the sick and unnecessary cells.
This was not done with anger or fear. It was
done in the same way her body knew how to
rid itself of used, unnecessary products. She
talked to the cells and, being a dancer, she
danced with them. She started using a castor
oil pack four times a week over her liver area
for an hour to an hour-and-a-half. She used
this time for meditation, visualizing the castor
oil as the healing power of the Palma Christi,
or the Palm of Christ. She had always eaten a
good diet, which she maintained, and she was
able to get acupuncture. She knew how to
work with her dreams and had followed their
guidance for many years. So this healing regimen was easy for her to apply to this situation.
After months of using the castor oil pack, she
no longer had the severe pain and her feeling
of well-being returned. She needed phleboto-
mies, at first, about every six weeks. When I
saw her this time, however, it had been four-
and-a-half months since she had needed one!
She's now in her late-70's and feels healthy
and well, although the diagnosis of polycythe-
mia rubra vera is still an issue that she has to
deal with. She told me during a visit in 2013
that people ask her about the disease. She
said she tries to explain it but doesn't know*

very much about it and doesn't find herself motivated to do an in-depth study of the disease itself. I found her comment to be very helpful and important in her healing. It is not her job to concentrate on her illness. Her job is to live her life, while I as her physician—along with her other physicians—need to understand and study the disease. The beauty of this lady is that she can continue with her love of life and her ability give light to other people's lives. She has not become her disease. **She happens to have the disease, but she is not the disease.** *She and her husband have moved into a new home that is easier to maintain. She sees this as a metaphor, and she is as busy redesigning her new home as she is in redesigning her physical body. I have heard it said that the new image of humanity emerging in our century is that of the Divine Artist in everyone. I believe that this wonderful lady is a prototype of the emerging Divine Human. We can all learn from her how to deal with health issues that arise: doing what we can to mitigate the disease process and not allowing ourselves to be overcome by the diagnosis or the prognosis.*

A *different* nursery rhyme represents Living Medicine: "Mary had a little lamb, whose fleece was white as snow, and everywhere that Mary went, that lamb was sure to go. It followed her to school one day, which was against the rule. It made the children laugh and play to see a lamb at school." Mary represents the healing, nurturing, feminine energy of medicine that is young and vibrant and very much alive, *unlike* the old woman. The little lamb represents the healing Life

Force within *each one* of us—the Physician Within. That lamb is so full of life that it wants to laugh and play, because it is bursting with its own *living* essence. It is also as *pure* as new-fallen snow, *not* toxic or contaminated. This lamb follows Mary into the School of Life, where all the problems that the child (or the child within *each* of us) faces. As students enter our medical schools, they bring with them their own "little lamb," which is the young, vibrant, nurturing, *feminine* energy of medicine. (*All* medical students, both male and female, are represented in this analogy by Mary). In Living Medicine, even though the students encounter the *conventional* way of dealing with disease, they *also* learn to *play* with the lamb. Issues are dealt with as diseases and problems are faced, instead of being beaten into submission and "put to bed." Issues are worked with and understood in a joyful, creative way that makes 'the children laugh and play." Mary also takes her lamb to school. To be *fully* effective as physicians committed to *true* healing, we must now take Living Medicine into the medical schools.

The Bible is filled with admonitions to remain joyful and tells us that **laughter heals**. I learned these important lessons a few years ago while driving my car home from work. I was really fussing at God during a very difficult time in my life when I was trying to understand what was happening. Suddenly, my mind was filled with the quotation: "This is the day the Lord hath made. Let us rejoice and be glad in it" (Psalm 118:24). I stopped my car, got out, stood beside it and said: "That's right. I'll be glad in it." I immediately knew that I had to change my license plate, which now reads "BEGLAD." Since then, every time I get into my car, I am reminded that it was *not* by chance that my parents named me Gladys. Perhaps one of the most important things I can do in this lifetime is to BE GLAD. This principle has been demonstrated *repeatedly* in my life since then, and in the most mundane of situations, as the following story illustrates.

I had been working with a group of people who were members of the staff at the Mayo Clinic in Phoenix. Twice before I had had the opportunity to speak from the podium in their main lecture hall. Their PA system was the best I had experienced in any other setting. No matter where I moved around the podium, it picked up my voice. On this occasion, I was giving a workshop and we were in a classroom instead of the lecture hall, so the PA system was completely different. The person who introduced me had trouble with the microphone, and so did I. The microphone did *not* pick up our voices, and we *each* twisted and turned it, yet neither of us could get it to work. Finally, one of the participants in the workshop who was familiar with this *specific* PA system came up to the podium and saw that *we were talking into the* podium light *and* not *the microphone!* This realization struck us all as so funny that everyone doubled up with laughter! In my experience, nothing is more helpful when we are teaching than to be able to start with a joke or, in this case, an actual humorous situation that the Universe provided.

After a trip to Japan where my daughter (Analea) and I had spent time teaching, one of the things we experienced and talked about was the reality that **laughter and a smile represents the one truly universal** language. People may not understand the words we are saying. However, they know and understand laughter. *It brings all races together at a level that crosses all barriers.* Our sense of humor may be different, yet what laughter does *for* and *to* us *all* is the same. **The healing power of laughter has been studied and proven to be a mighty force.** Years ago, the breakthrough study on this topic was published by Norman Cousins[207] (1915-1990*).* He forged an unusual collaboration with his physician when he was diagnosed with a crippling and irreversible disease. *Together* they beat the odds, and Cousins was able to overcome his terminal illness by simply watching comedy and laughing, hour after hour. There have been many research studies done since the publication of this landmark book to validate and corroborate Cousins' experience.[208]

Anger, resentment, fear and other negative emotions reside in the adrenals (third chakra). At the same time, the adrenals represent

---

[207] Cousins, Norman. Anatomy of an Illness as Perceived by the Patient, 1979 (20th Anniversary Edition, 2005).

[208] https://www.ncbi.nlm.nih.gov>pubmed>PMID31488780.

a powerful center where forgiveness can *transform* these negative emotions into a positive force. We know that the adrenals can be activated by physical jolting, such as athletes do when they "pump their adrenals" by forcing their energy up along their back as their heels hit the ground. Hitler used this concept with his army when they marched and did the "goose step," a way of marching where their heels hit the ground in a forceful manner. Every time this happened, the soldier jolted his adrenals and activated the fighting Spirit within himself. If a person is in a competition or getting ready for battle, whether on the playing field or on an *actual* battlefield, the physical stimulation of the adrenals activates a physical process within the body. In so doing, one becomes a better fighter. *When a person laughs, it is almost impossible to fight.* While pumping the adrenals activates the *forceful* aspect of the adrenals, laughter literally "tickles" the adrenals. As we laugh, our diaphragm bounces up and down. The adrenals, which sit directly underneath the diaphragm, get gently activated by a rhythmic pulsation. That energy then moves up from the adrenals into the heart (fourth chakra or the love center). When a person is laughing, it is impossible to march! With *hilarious* laughter, it is almost impossible to stand up. With *healing* laughter, it is almost impossible not to forgive. *Forgiveness and laughter go hand in hand and are the outcome of love.* **So,** let us remember that **no matter how hard our lives are or how many difficulties we find ourselves in, these *can* and *will be* overcome, if we allow ourselves to "rejoice" and let laughter do its healing magic.**

Let the playroom in our Living Medicine dwelling place become filled with the *music* of our choice, with *beauty* that we appreciate and with *laughter* that stimulates and activates our Life Force. Then, with the very loving essence of the healing heart, the playroom *also* becomes a place within our Living Medicine home where we can be healed.

8

The Bathroom

In our house of Living Medicine, the bathroom is a place for cleansing, elimination, grooming and privacy. *Every cell* of our body needs to be able to *take in nutrients* and assimilate them. If they cannot, the body will die from starvation. By the same token, if our cells are unable to eliminate the byproducts of their own metabolism, the body will also die. This is why IV nutrients, feeding tubes, colostomy bags and kidney dialysis are considered to be lifesaving (or life-sustaining) treatments for the *physical* body in conventional medicine. Living Medicine physicians, however, believe that **assimilation and elimination in *all* aspects of our being are *essential* to life.** The more we physicians can help patients understand *in their own terms* the importance of this process, the more they will be able to accept *their* role in keeping this vital aspect of their physiology functioning well.

In Israel, the Jordan River starts in the higher regions of Mount Hermon and flows down into the Sea of Galilee. Birds fly over this sea, fish live in it, and people live and flowers grow all around it. *It is a very living, active sea.* This *same* water then travels down and empties into the Dead Sea. *Nothing* lives or grows in the Dead Sea. *No one* can live around it. Birds will *not* fly over it and plants do *not* grow around it. *The only difference* between the Sea of Galilee and the Dead Sea is that *the latter has no way of eliminating or allowing for run off, as it has no outlet.* This fact, then, becomes the metaphor for the bathroom in our Living Medicine dwelling place.

On a *physical* level, we have many examples of this Sea of Galilee/ Dead Sea phenomenon. For example, in the RESPIRATORY system, we *take in* oxygen (O2) and *must be able to eliminate* carbon dioxide (CO2). Anything that interferes with this process causes illness and, ultimately, death. The same is true of Mother Earth's respiratory system, only in reverse: she needs our CO2 to be able to give us our O2. Because we have allowed the air on this planet to become polluted, *we inhale all manner of substances that are not conducive to* our *good health*, nor Mother Earth's. (Interestingly though, with the global pandemic of 2020 requiring "sheltering in place" in the majority of the world, the air has cleared up so much that *Mother Earth can now breathe* better than she has been able to breathe for over thirty years! As a result, I can also *now* see the Himalayas in photographs as I saw them as a child.)

In the ALIMENTARY CANAL, food *must* be digested and processed, and the waste *must* be eliminated. If anything interferes with this process, we become sick and can die. Likewise, in the URINARY SYSTEM, the liquids that we take in are channeled through the kidneys, processed through the urinary tract and then eliminated. Any interference with this process causes illness and can also lead to death.

Because the LYMPHATIC SYSTEM *is truly the "waste management" system of the body*, the example of the Sea of Galilee/Dead Sea phenomenon is even more evident in this system. The body's lymph vessels surround *every* cell and play an essential part in delivering nutrients to *each* cell and removing the *unusable* metabolic byproducts. *If too many byproducts and toxins accumulate in the lymphatic system, impairing the natural intake and outflow, the cells will die.* One of the reasons **castor oil is** so **effective in** the healing process is that it is *absorbed* by the lymphatics of the skin and then carried to the *deeper* lymphatics, **helping to keep the lymph clean**. It is like rain in the mountains. The rain (castor oil) comes down between the rocks, goes into little rivulets (lymphatic vessels), then into pools (lymph nodes) that flow into larger streams (lymphatic ducts) and rivers (the subclavian veins). Ultimately, the byproducts of metabolism are carried by the lymphatic fluid out into the ocean (the body's ELIMINATION SYSTEM: colon, kidneys, lungs and skin). Thus, whatever else castor oil does, it certainly serves a vital role in the cleansing process associated with the lymphatic system.

When it comes to understanding the process of elimination in the body, sometimes a picture is worth a thousand words! That is why I asked Dr. Ann to include the following handouts[209] that she uses with her patients to help them understand this important process. In her opinion, these "pictures" are especially helpful in teaching her patients the importance of eliminating *toxic waste* from the body. An explanation of the handouts follows.

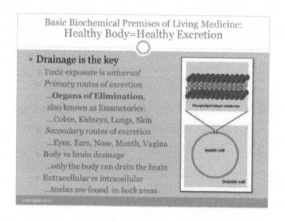

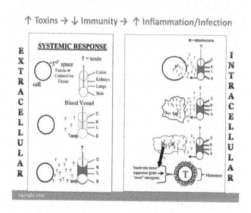

---

[209] McCombs, Ann, DO. Text written by Dr. Ann in 1999 and 2012 and original artwork commissioned by her, ©2012.

The *first diagram* is simply a pictorial illustration of the Sea of Galilee/Dead Sea phenomenon previously described.

The *second diagram* illustrates the *progression of toxic waste accumulation*, if it is not eliminated in a timely way. In the *extracellular* space (the space *outside* the cell), *healthy* elimination is demonstrated by the left uppermost picture: toxins come into our system and easily exit through the *primary* organs of elimination: *colon, kidneys, lungs and skin*. This process is accomplished with the help of our lymphatic system as explained above. If toxic material is not or cannot be eliminated in a timely way, it continues to accumulate. It is pushed from the circulatory system (represented by the blood vessel in this diagram) *deeper* into the tissues in a *sequential* way:

- Into the *connective tissue* (fascia or "third space")— the middle illustration on the left—often seen symptomatically as an *acute* allergic reaction, since the toxin is a "foreign" substance that the body knows doesn't belong there;
- then towards the cell itself—the lower illustration on the left— as the third space becomes more and more filled with toxic material, usually experienced as a *chronic* allergic reaction;
- once the third space is *completely* full, the toxic waste is driven into the cell (*intracellular* space)—the upper illustration on the right—symptomatically manifesting now as *fatigue* (tired/ low energy, often with little to no motivation to do much of anything), because the toxin has "attacked" the mitochondria (the part of the cell that generates the energy of the body);
- when the mitochondria get overwhelmed by the toxic waste and the cell's DNA (genetic material) is "attacked" next by the invasion of toxins —the middle illustration on the right—the energy of the body becomes depleted in a *major* way, symptomatically observed as *chronic* fatigue (energy is so low that the patient can hardly get out of bed and finds him/herself sleeping sixteen or more hours a day);

- lastly, if *effective* elimination becomes impossible, the DNA of the cell will be destroyed, and the toxin then fills up the cell *completely*—the lower illustration on the right—now symptomatically manifesting as *cancer* (benign or malignant). This dying cell will then do all it can to wall itself off from the rest of its neighboring cells to keep the toxic waste from spreading into other cells. In its wisdom, this cell is really making a decision to sacrifice itself, in a sense, for the good of the *whole* body.

In summary, *any* kind of metabolic waste can become toxic (like the Dead Sea) if it is not *effectively* eliminated from the body in a healthy and timely way. The *simplest* way to create "natural" elimination is to:

- Breathe *clean* air, if you can (using a HEPA filter on your furnace is ideal or make sure your room air purifier has one in it);
- drink *clean* water, if available— otherwise, boil the water you have access to ("structured" water is the *best* option, in Dr. Ann's opinion, which will be discussed later in this chapter);
- eat *clean* food (organic, if possible, no matter what dietary regimen you choose); and use a *castor oil pack* as directed in the references given in chapter five.

Other ways of detoxing the body are certainly available and *may* need to be employed. We think *simple* prevention is best, however, if at all possible.

The *respiratory system* is also important for reasons other than the *physical* elimination of toxic waste. Whether we are awake or asleep, conscious or unconscious, *as long as we are alive, we breathe*. We can live longer without food or water than we can live without breathing air. Yet, because breathing is so natural to us and so essential to life on this planet, most of us remain *unaware* of our breath. Not being attuned to what it means to *really* breathe, we mostly just breathe to maintain life and do not TRULY *breathe*. In God's scheme of things, breath was *essential* for humankind to become a *living* being. All the great religious and spiritual disciplines have been aware of how important breath is, and they incorporate *conscious* breathing into their physical practices. Thus, it seems reasonable that, *as we become more* conscious *of our breath, we also become more conscious of our spiritual being-ness*.

Breathing is, in fact, critically important in *every* aspect of our lives, as *each* cell in our body requires oxygen to maintain its life and will die if deprived of it for even a short amount of time (three to six minutes). Two examples come to mind. As I have watched the great athletes in the Summer Olympics over the years, I noticed how aware they were of their breath and their control of it. They knew that to be in control of their body and their mind, breathing had to be coordinated and in tune with *all* their actions. Likewise, when I was assisting pregnant women in birthing their babies, one of the first things we taught the mother-to-be was *how to breathe with her contractions*, since oxygen is so vital to her and her baby. The baby needs the oxygen that the mother breathes *in* to ensure its proper growth during the pregnancy. During labor, when contractions are long and hard, the baby's need for oxygen becomes *even more* significant. If the mother does not get enough oxygen to the baby, severe problems can occur. The mother also needs oxygen to be able to maintain *her* muscle contractions during labor. In addition, **the *way* the mother breathes—and the *consciousness* she maintains *as* she breathes—allows her to move into and through the pain of labor.** *The more control she has over her breathing, the more control she has over the labor itself.* The progress of labor is thus significantly enhanced or impeded by the way the mother breathes.

Dr. Ann has a third example from her medical training that also demonstrates the importance of the breath. As a third-year medical student, she was doing her *first* surgical clinical rotation with a general surgeon. One of his specialties was using the gastric balloon procedure to help morbidly obese patients achieve weight loss (a precursor to the current procedure of gastric band surgery). On this particular day, the surgeon was scheduled to take out one of these gastric balloons emergently and was having difficulty doing so. As he kept trying and failing to get it out, he was becoming more and more frustrated. Dr. Ann suggested that he try using the patient's breathing to assist with the removal of the gastric balloon. He had no idea what she meant. As she began to explain her idea to him, he threw his instruments down on the surgical tray and said: "If you think that will work, then *you* do it!" and walked away from the surgery table. Though shocked by the surgeon's behavior and feeling very scared, she picked up the instruments and was able to gently and easily remove the gastric balloon, little by little, every time the patient exhaled (breathed out). They later discussed what happened in the operating room in his office. He asked her how she knew to try that technique. She explained her training in OMT and how a patient's breathing is often used to assist with certain techniques. Unbeknownst to her at the time, as a result of that experience and many others while using osteopathic principles and practices during her surgical rotation with him, he gave her the highest score for her surgical rotation that he had *ever* given a medical student! They also became friends and enjoyed a warm collegial relationship from that time on while she was at that hospital. This change in behavior greatly surprised the hospital staff, especially the operating room nurses, as this physician had a reputation for being very difficult to work with and for having little to no bedside manner.

I have found in my practice of medicine that many of my patients who suffer from various illnesses, including depression and fatigue, are *unaware* of their breathing; sometimes to the extent that they hardly breathe at all. They often use only the *upper* part of their lungs to make the exchange of air, which is just barely enough to allow them to survive. As I listen to their chest and ask them to breathe deeply, very often the breath sounds do not extend below the shoulder blades. This means that the exchange of oxygen occurs only in the *upper* part of the lungs. The *residual* air in their lungs does *not* have a good oxygen-carbon dioxide exchange ratio. As we discuss their breathing, patients become more aware of what it feels like to have a breath that goes *deep* into their lungs to rid the lungs of accumulated residual air. They begin to feel better, and their health improves. *Controlled breathing is a great stress reducer. It also allows oxygen to get to the brain and nervous system, as well as into the muscular system of the body.* In this way, *oxygen* can greatly reduce muscle spasms and tension, *far* better than prescribing a muscle relaxer or Valium! I suggest to my patients that they *consciously* breathe *in* joy and breathe *out* fear, breathe *in* energy and breathe *out* fatigue, breathe *in* laughter and breathe *out* anger, etc. I recommend that they do this several times a day, for short periods of time. I also propose that they *consciously* inhale into their physical being whatever spiritual quality they are looking for, then *consciously* exhale to rid themselves of whatever negative aspects of their being that they are ready to release. **I know of no disease process, whether it be physical, mental, emotional or spiritual, that is not helped on its path toward healing by *conscious* breathing.** It takes so little time, it is a hundred percent free and an available resource 24/7, no matter *what* physical condition a person is in. In addition, no one and nothing else can breathe *for* us (unless we are on a ventilator). I truly believe that *if each one of us would do some active* conscious *breathing, this whole planet would be a better place in which to live.*

In the UROGENITAL SYSTEM, when there is *improper* elimination, women can suffer from problems such as *dysmenorrhea*—painful menstruation that is *not* a disease, is *not* fatal and does *not* affect all women. It is, however, a problem that, for hundreds of years, has caused severe pain and discomfort. Many women are unable to work from one to seven days a month due to the pain and discomfort from their menstrual periods. For some women, this condition severely limits their ability to function *at all*. When I started practicing medicine, very little was known about ways in which to alleviate this condition. Conventional medicine has given us *some* tools to help with the problem. Some women have even been given strong narcotics to help them deal with their pain. Unfortunately, some of these medications completely stop *all* menstruation. I am concerned about our interference with this *natural* process. However, I recognize that pain medication *may* be needed in some instances until the root cause of that degree of discomfort can be evaluated, treated and resolved.

The causes of dysmenorrhea are numerous. *In young girls*, an immature uterus, a small cervical opening, endometriosis, a retroverted or tilted uterus or other *structural* problems with the female organs can *all* contribute to this condition. Poor posture, nutritional deficiencies, trauma and psychological problems can also be causative factors. *In mature women*, uterine fibroids, endometriosis, abdominal adhesions, pelvic inflammatory disease, ovarian tumors, bowel conditions, as well as structural problems, can also be contributory to dysmenorrhea. Some doctors now realize that a lack of *healthy* nutrition can be a major factor as well. Young women who are trying to maintain an *extremely* thin body can have severe problems as a result of not eating well, especially if they are anorexic or bulimic. On the other hand, problems such as hypothyroidism, pituitary dysfunction, adrenal insufficiency and even obesity can *also* cause difficulties with menstrual problems. Plenty of *clean* water, a BALANCED DIET with *natural* foods, *fresh* fruits and vegetables, *moderate* amounts of *dairy* products, and plenty of *fiber*— which eliminates the tendency towards constipation, are all helpful adjuncts as well. Excess intake of simple carbohydrates, *especially* refined *sugar*, can be particularly detrimental around the time of the menstrual period. Exercise is likewise extremely important. A woman who is sitting at a desk all day is more apt to have difficulty with her periods, partly because of lymphatic congestion in the pelvic area. *Activity* helps to diminish this, e.g. walking, bicycle riding, swimming and dancing. *Too much* strenuous activity, however, can cause muscle strain and sprain, and even amenorrhea (absence of the menstrual period), so it is *not* recommended. At the risk of being redundant, we cannot emphasize how important it is to get *enough* rest and *alleviate stress* as much as possible.

Regular osteopathic or chiropractic adjustments also make good sense when treating dysmenorrhea, since any neurological, muscular or structural dysfunction can aggravate this condition. I have found that the use of a castor oil pack during the menstrual period can also provide relief, as well as comfort, to those who suffer from this condition. When women start experiencing menstrual discomfort, they can take the castor oil pack—along with their hot water bottle or heating pad—and place it on their major area of discomfort. Then, they simply lie down and allow themselves to relax. Frequently, doing just this little bit of *cost-effective intervention* will cause the pain to ease off. Castor oil packs can also be used *preventatively* on a monthly basis, for three consecutive days each week. *For some women, this simple, non-toxic, cost-effective therapy can eliminate their menstrual problems altogether.* Castor oil packs help ease lymphatic congestion, venous stasis, muscle tension and inflammation in general. In my experience, women who have used the castor oil pack for small uterine fibroids frequently have been able to eliminate them completely, and *some* ovarian cysts have also responded well to castor oil pack therapy.

Attitudes and emotions are also very closely linked to dysmenorrhea. When a young girl is told to just "get over it" or "tough it out," these words can cause serious trauma that can last a lifetime. On the other hand, if some *mild* discomfort gets the attention she is looking for, her discomfort can become a way she can gain the attention she is needing. However, I have found that the *fear* of impending pain that some women live with, month after month, can be devastating. In addition, **if sexual abuse is a factor in her dysmenorrhea, it must be addressed.**

Those of us who live in the desert are *very* aware of how important it is to get *enough* water into our systems for our overall health. Like all other organs of the body, the proper functioning of *all* emunctories (organs of elimination) relies on the steady inflow and outflow of water in *every* cell of our body.[210,211] As it turns out, however, the *kind*

---

[210] Pollack, Gerald H. Cells, Gels and the Engines of Life, 2001.

[211] Pollack, Gerald H. et.al. (editors). Water and the Cell, 2006.

of water we take into our bodies also makes an *enormous* difference in how well these metabolic processes function. This is a fact I have both learned and personally experienced the value of within the past year from Dr. Ann. We have both been using *structured water*, also known as "the fourth phase of water," a hydrator that both of us have *greatly* benefitted from, and one that Dr. Gerald Pollack has been researching for many years.[212] This kind of water creates a "double-double- helix" (a double-helix inside of a double-helix) and "nanosizes" the water molecules (makes them *extremely* tiny). Nutrients can then go *into* the cell and toxins and metabolic waste can also be eliminated *from* the cell much more quickly, efficiently and effectively. Dr. Ann has also observed the tremendous difference structured water has made in the veteran population she works with at the Warrior Healing Center in Sierra Vista, Arizona. In her opinion, as a "rogue scientist who thinks outside-the-box," Dr. Pollack may just be the best example of Albert Szent-Györgyi's classic definition of research: "...to see what everybody has seen and think what nobody has thought" (paraphrased from the German philosopher, Arthur Schopenhauer).[213]

Only certain organs in the body have the capacity to regenerate themselves to full function, and none of our urogenital organs can do that...*yet*. With the advent of stem cell therapy and 3-D printing, however, who knows what *may* be possible in the human body in the years to come?

In the *conventional* medical model, *physical* elimination is what is predominantly emphasized. It is just as important, however, to keep the elimination flowing on the mental, emotional and spiritual levels as well. **Mentally, if we do not use what we have learned, we lose our ability to access information and learn from it.** For example, I know a registered nurse who has degrees in psychology and *many* teaching certificates. She continually goes to school, learning more and more, yet *uses* very little of her knowledge in practice. In fact, when a subject is raised in conversational circles, she does *not* have

---

[212] Pollack, Gerald H. The Fourth Phase of Water: Beyond Solid, Liquid, Vapor, 2013.
[213] www.quoteinvestigator.com>2015/07/04.

a great deal to contribute. However, I have other friends who have only *minimal* educational opportunities who strive *every day* to use everything they have *ever* learned in their lives. They understand the importance of "use it or lose it," so they *eagerly share* their knowledge with, and are willing to learn from, other people. When engaged in a conversation, they usually have something to say on almost *any* subject. Their knowledge is *not* stuck someplace in their mind. It is *readily accessible information* to them because they constantly *use* it.

On the *emotional* level, we are constantly being challenged to choose what to hold onto and what to let go of. Sometimes, we must become quite creative in how to do this in our lives. We have available to us the *choice* between what is valuable and what is "excess baggage." I found myself having to make such a choice after my divorce. For years, the pain I felt from this experience remained so *acute* that my involvement in the pain was a *daily* struggle. I worked on forgiveness. However, that choice just did not seem accessible to me until I decided I had to FIRST *live through* the pain of betrayal and loss. Once I could do that, I could move into an awareness of what I had really *gained* from my marriage and the life I had lived up to that point. I finally realized that *I* had the choice of what I really wanted to continue to live with. What I realized was that I had enjoyed forty-six years of a marriage that *I* considered fulfilling and loving. The work that we had done *together*, the children we had raised, the lives we had touched, the joy that we had shared and the experiences that we had created and developed were *all* available to me in my memory. *My love for what had been was a living thing,* because it brought joy to my heart, a smile to my face and continued to enrich the life I was subsequently living. I could then look at my ex-husband in a *loving* way and thank him for giving me the opportunity to share his life. I came to understand that **the process of forgiveness is also a *living* thing.** *Although I still felt the pain of what "might have been," it became a bittersweet pain, instead of a deadly, consuming one.* I realized that the statement: "It's better to have loved and lost than never to have loved at all" had *real* depth and truth to it. When we choose Life and let go of those things that have burdened us, we transform our *experience* of life and living.

In looking back on my life experiences, I have become aware that the ones I had that were hurtful and painful are *now* like scars that have healed over. They no longer hold the pain that they held at the time they were created. I can look back and say: "Oh, that was a really hard and painful time." However, I no longer have the *feeling* of pain that accompanies that memory. When I look back on my memories that were joyful and pleasant, I remember them and can feel the joy, love and excitement that went with them. **The painful times leave scars. The joyful and good times become *living* memories that *still* bring joy and hope.** Perhaps an indication of how we are progressing on this emotional path is to look back and see which of our memories *still* have feelings associated with them. If we have painful memories that are *still* alive, it may be that it is like having an injury and continually picking at the scab. The injury then does *not* heal. However, by allowing that injury to heal with time, it simply becomes a scar that we can run our finger over, remembering what happened, yet no longer have any *painful* feelings associated with it.

It is also important to understand this concept of healing on *every* level. For example, on a *physical* level, if we have an abscess, there is severe pain until it is drained. On an *emotional* level, if we try to hang onto the love of a person who has already moved on, the pain becomes that of a broken heart. On the *mental* level, if we have concepts of ideology or theology that no longer serve us as our knowledge grows and our understanding evolves, then the ensuing mental conflict can cause severe distress. On the *spiritual* level, if we try to hang onto our experience of God from the past as an angry God, we may feel separated from the God that gave us Life and Love. This separation becomes an experience of what has been called the "dark night of the soul." We can transform this darkness, however, as we move through it into the light. *We can experience a living, loving and forgiving God once we let go of the angry one.* As long as we perceive the concept of an angry God as being *right* for us, it is a concept that is still in the light. When we embrace a *different* concept of God and move on, our *previous* concept of God then seems *dark* to us. Another example of this concept is how the parts of our "shadow self" seem dark before they move from the unconscious (darkness) into the conscious (light). I realize that some of these concepts may seem "heady" and perhaps difficult to fully grasp at first glance. I trust that the following story about my brother Carl's patient in Nepal will bring these concepts into clearer focus and understanding.

Carl received his MD degree from Harvard in the early 1940's and worked with my parents during the partition of India. They used a mobile medical unit to travel around, helping the Hindus and Moham-medans who were moving from their homes to another part of India. The soul of India was being torn apart during this time, and the suffer-ing was unimaginable. Shortly after this incredible turmoil—on *every* level—in India ended on August 15, 1947, Carl was invited to be the physician for the team sponsored by National Geographic to photo-graph the birds of Nepal. The team was headed by Robert Fleming, a family friend and professor at Woodstock, the school in the Himalayas where we children had all been educated. The team traveled by foot for six weeks, climbing up and down the Himalayan Mountains. When the Nepalese people heard that there was a doctor with the team, they would gather at the team's campsite, looking for medical help.

One day a man was brought to the campsite, having been car-ried by his friends on a stretcher. When Carl saw him, he realized *immediately* that this man was terminally ill. His arms and legs were just skin and bones, and his abdomen was *severely* swollen. Carl told the people who brought the man that he really did not know what he could do for him. He had no equipment with him to deal with this sort of problem. The man's friends said to Carl: "We have walked for two days to bring this man here. You're a doctor, aren't you?" My brother took a deep breath and said: "Yes, I am," realizing that he really had to do *something* for this man. Carl's diagnosis was that the man had developed a severe amoebic abscess and that the only thing he could do for him to give him *any* relief would be to drain that abscess. He only had a small Boy Scout knife with him. He made an incision in the man's abdomen and drained *two buckets* of pus from his swollen belly. Because he and the team were leaving the next day, Carl knew that he had to put *some* type of drain into the incision that he had just made in this man's abdomen. If he did not do this, it would continue to drain *or* the incision would close and the abscess process would continue, likely resulting in the man's death. Carl had nothing with him to use as a drain, so he cut about an inch off the end of the tubing of his stethoscope and stitched that into the man's incision. The team left as scheduled the next day. Carl heard nothing from this man or the village after that day. *He had no idea whether this man had lived or died.*

Twenty-five years later, Carl decided to take his children and some of his grandchildren to Nepal to repeat the National Geographic trek. They traveled for six weeks, retracing the steps of Carl's earlier journey, having a wonderful time doing so. When the family came to the place where Carl had treated this patient, he stopped to tell his children the *amazing* story of this very ill Nepalese man. The hill people had gathered around, as was the custom when visitors arrived in the area. A man came up to Carl to ask if he recognized him. Carl had *no* recollection of ever meeting this man before. Nevertheless, the man was smiling broadly and, with a great deal of joy, told Carl that HE *was the man whose abdomen Carl had incised and drained twenty-five years ago!* Now here he was, standing *directly* in front of Carl, happy and healthy!

Two important principles are illustrated by this story: Even if we physicians *don't* have the sophisticated tools and equipment that we were trained with and have learned to depend on, **we must never forget the oath we all took: "*First*, do no harm."** No matter what conditions or circumstances our patients present to us, as physicians we will always be *expected* to bring *some* form of relief to those who seek our help. If we are striving to do *our own* healing work on *every* level, we can rest assured and trust that *something* will come to us in the moment to do for our patients to relieve their suffering. It could be a makeshift drain made with a Boy Scout knife to keep an incision open, like Carl did, or a simple healing touch and a compassionate listening ear. If we *have not yet* taken the time to do that kind of *personal* growth work in our lives, we may just find ourselves feeling helpless and clueless in those moments. Then we will miss the opportunities our patients present to us *every day* to help them *truly* heal. *No matter what we do for our patients, though,* **if we offer what we can with a** **loving** **heart, an** **open** **mind and create the experience of being** **truly and deeply listened to,** **SOME aspect of healing will** *always* **be possible**.

There is an old proverb that says: "As a man thinketh in his heart, so is he" (Proverbs 23:7). Two other wise sayings from the Cayce material are: "Thoughts are things"[214] and "Spirit is the life, mind is the builder and physical is the result."[215] **If we hang onto thoughts and** **become so convinced that** *certain* **ones are true, they** *become* **real in our physical body.** This concept was demonstrated to me years ago when an eighty-four-year-old woman came into my office suffering from a severe respiratory problem. She greeted me with the words: "I haven't seen a doctor for sixty-seven years. I don't like doctors, and you're not going to put me in the hospital." Well, *that* is an interesting way to be greeted by a patient and sets the boundaries very clearly! I accepted her terms and said: "Okay. *Now* what can I do for you?" She reported that she was having trouble breathing and was also experiencing chest pains. I examined and listened to her chest and, sure enough, she had full-blown pneumonia that could be treated medically, and I told her so. In the process of my examining her, I saw and felt a mass in her left breast larger than a golf ball. When I touched it, I *knew* it was cancer. I asked her: "How long have you had this in your breast?" She replied: "Ten years." I said: "Oh, really? What have you done about it?" She said: "Well, when I look at it and I see that it's growing, I say to it: 'Stop it!' and it stops for a while. And we go on, and it's just there, and nothing happens until it decides to grow again, and I tell it to 'stop it' again. I've been able to keep it

---

[214] www.edgarcayce.org. Reading 1581-1.

[215] www.edgarcayce.org. Reading 900-70.

at this size now for ten years. It doesn't hurt, it's just there." So, I said to her: "Have you ever thought about trying to make it go away?" Her response was: "No. How would I do that?" I explained some of the concepts of visualization to her. I shared with her how, when people visualize their white blood cells working *with* cancer cells, they sometimes engulf the cancer cells, allowing the healing process to start. She liked that idea. She is a woman whose body knew what she meant when she said: "Stop it!" and it stopped whatever she told it to and whenever she told it to. She left my office, and I did not see her for another six months. When she returned, the lesion had reduced itself by a full centimeter! I said: "Wow! That's great. Now are you going to keep it up?" She said: "Yes." So, for another six months, she worked on it. When she came back again, it was even smaller. Then, I did not see her for two years. When I did see her again, the breast mass was the same size as it had been when I had seen her two years earlier. I said: "What happened?" Her comment was: "Oh, I got tired of fussing with that old thing. You know, it's never going to kill me." And you know what? I knew that it *never* would! *She and that cancer were living so comfortably together that it wouldn't* dare *kill her!* Someday, she may trip and fall down the stairs and die. However, she will *not* die from *that* cancer! There are many people who, when they die and their bodies are autopsied, are found to have cancers that they had lived with compatibly *for many years*, as their autopsies revealed that they had died of some *totally unrelated* problem.[216]

I believe that we physicians have done a great disservice to our patients by telling them to check for lumps in their breasts every month. In so doing, I think we may be planting *recurring* seeds of their *fear* of finding cancer, especially when *we* help them visualize what to look for. We tell them in *great detail* how to do this monthly check by diagraming it for them and even drawing pictures of what they are to look for. Perhaps we should instead be teaching our patients to stand in front of the mirror each month and appreciate

---

[216] Karwinski, B. et.al., "Clinically undiagnosed malignant tumours found at autopsy," https://doi.org/10.1111/j.16990463.1990.tb01062.x.

the *beauty* of their body, thanking God for the functionality of it. During that time, perhaps we should encourage them to *appreciate* their breasts for the nurturing that comes from them, recalling the *collective comfort* each one of our species has received from our mothers' breasts throughout time. By asking the patients in our practices to check each month for the presence of a potentially fatal diagnosis, their breasts have now become their *enemy* as they "check them for lumps." I'm certain that *all* physicians now have patients (both female *and* male, since breast cancer in men is now a statistic we must also pay attention to) who are afraid to touch their breasts for fear they will find lumps. We also have patients who check and check until they finally find something. It is as if the body's response to this monthly "fear check" says: "Oh, you're looking for lumps? Well, let me give you one or two." By encouraging this monthly ritual in the name of prevention, I think we have planted *time bombs* in our beautiful bodies. Instead of standing in front of our bathroom mirror and thanking God for this magnificent body that He has given us (no matter what its shape), *we look for the worst*. Why can't we change that? Why can't we look at ourselves, see our breasts and say something like: "Hello, there! How are you? Do you have a message for me?" and learn to check our breasts with appreciation? By approaching a *routine* breast self-exam in this more upbeat and *neutral* way, our bodies can then let us know if there *is* an issue. *If* there is an issue that needs to be dealt with, we will know it because our bodies will tell us. **The Physician Within *each* one of us *knows* if there is a problem and, if so, *what* to look for, *how* to look for it and how to get our attention so we can become *aware* of it.** My own journey through breast cancer diagnosis and treatment which follows is a good example of this important principle.

A few years ago, my son (Bob) asked me to speak at one of the Human Potential Center conferences in Austin, Texas. I was delighted to do this, and we had a great conference. I spoke to a crowd of probably two hundred people. As part of my talk, I told them my thoughts on how we physicians typically deal with breast cancer in our society (recapped in the previous paragraph). At the end of my talk, I reiterated the statement: "Your body will know if there's a problem, and it will let you know." When I came home from Austin and was digging in my garden two months later, a shovel handle bumped me *hard* in my left breast. I developed a large hematoma there. With the use of arnica and castor oil packs over the next several weeks, however, it almost went away...but not quite. There was still something there in my left breast which did not feel right. So, I decided to do a mammogram. Sure enough, it showed that calcifications indicative of the presence of cancer were present in one small lump. I had a biopsy done of the lump which validated what I suspected: breast cancer. When I heard this diagnosis, I *immediately* decided that *I* did not have cancer...that what *I* had was a *lump in my left breast that had some cancer cells in it.*

I knew that there were many holistic techniques that I could do (on an *energetic* level, as well as on the *physical* level, including a variety of different dietary approaches) that could get rid of the cancer cells. At that time in my life, however, I was very busy and just *didn't have time* to pursue any of those holistic paths. I then realized I had *another* choice: I could have the lump removed! It was a simple procedure and available to me, so I made an appointment with a surgeon. We then set up a time to do the lumpectomy. I immediately started talking to my body, specifically to the area where the cancer cells were. *In my mind*, I created a beautiful little leather suitcase, all hand-tooled and made specifically for this work. I told the cancer cells that this little suitcase was for *them*. I invited them to come and get into the suitcase and bring with them any cancer cells which might be in any other part of my body. I told them they were going to have a family reunion, after which they were all going to take a trip together. On the day of the surgery, all those cells knew that this was *the* day they were going to be gone and leave my body. I was not angry with them or afraid of them. It was just time for them to leave.

After the surgery, there was still some question about the margins, so the surgeon recommended radiation. Through the years, in dealing with women who had breast cancer and had had radiation, I had seen the devastation and damage to the body that this treatment caused. I really questioned this recommendation. I also knew that the way radiation was being applied at the time of *my* diagnosis was quite different from what I had previously experienced with my patients. I knew I had to get more information, so I went to talk to the radiologist who would be doing the work, *if* I chose that path. This kind physician said to me: "Let me tell you a story. A few years ago, I was working with a colleague in New Orleans. We were researching ways in which radiation could be applied more specifically and in a more controlled way. One day, I had a woman come into the lab, and she had with her an entourage of people. She said to me: 'I'm the most important and wealthiest person in Argentina. I've had cancer removed from my breast, and I am to receive radiation therapy. I don't have time for this kind of treatment and will not accept radiation therapy that's going to injure more of my body. So, I'm here to tell you that I need you to find a way that I can receive the radiation therapy without damaging other parts of my body. I want you to find some way that will work for *my* body *specifically*.' It so happened that was *exactly* the kind of work that my colleague and I had been working on! We came up with a *specific* therapy for her that is now called *brachytherapy*. This kind of radiation therapy is directed *only* at the specific cells contained within the area of the tumor." This approach made sense to me and, with only five treatments, I was declared "cancer-free" and have had no problem since. What I learned from this experience is that *my* Physician Within knew *exactly* what *I* needed and *how* to help me find it... *and it did!*

I also want to mention here that both Dr. Ann and I have treated *many* individuals dealing with cancer over the years over the years. We have *both* observed that **cancer has a strong tendency to recur if the patient does not "get the message" about why the cancer occurred in the first place.** Dr. Ann learned this principle during her clinical rotations with Bernie Siegel, MD while attending his ECaP[217]

---

[217] www.berniesiegelmd.com.

groups for two months. I learned it when I dealt with my own experience of having cancer. There are many resources for addressing this issue, including the research of Lawrence LeShan, PhD[218] (who is almost three months older than I am, still alive and I trust, *also* "aging into health"!) and Gabor Maté, MD.[219]

The bathroom is the room in our Living Medicine dwelling place where we really *can* make friends with our bodies, our minds and our spirits. The bathroom is also a place where we can take healthful, invigorating showers or baths and wash our hair, letting tension and stress simply go down the drain. While hot baths are very helpful for *some* people in promoting relaxation and letting the muscles rejuvenate, for *other* people a warm shower may feel soothing and more to their liking. Thus, the bathroom becomes a place where *individual* needs and preferences can be honored.

If we have a bathroom where there is a bathtub, there are several things that will help us in *balancing* our body, mind and spirit. For example, when traveling for long distances, jet lag can be a problem. It can be alleviated by putting a cup of Epsom salts and a cup of baking soda in a tub of warm water (*not* too hot, just good and warm), then immersing ourselves fully in it for fifteen minutes or so (without crossing our legs or arms). On getting out of the tub (again, *without* crossing any body parts), dry off with a towel and get into bed. Rest or sleep for as long as possible, even if it is just an hour or so, before getting up and going on with your trip in your *new* time zone.

As a final point, in the bathroom, a mirror is usually present. What we see in the mirror is the reflection of how we see ourselves, *not* the way other people see us. Other people see us through *their* eyes, which actually reflects who and what *they* are. Alice in Wonderland went through the "looking glass" to get to the deeper parts of herself. This is the mirror through which we see the world *outside*

---

[218] LeShan, Lawrence, PhD. *You Can Fight For Your Life: Emotional Factors in the Treatment of Cancer,* 1980; and *Cancer as a Turning Point: A Handbook for People with Cancer, Their Families and Health Professionals,* 1989 and 1994 (revised ed.).

[219] Maté, Gabor, MD. *When the Body Says NO: Exploring the Stress-Disease Connection,* 2011.

of ourselves, as well as view those deeper parts *within* ourselves. **A disease process that can be diagnosed and treated from the *outside* by a physician can only be understood and *truly* healed IF the *inner* aspects of the patient are brought forth and allowed to manifest.** As the patient looks into the mirror and sees the reflection of what their disease process is saying to *them*, we begin to understand their disease in a way that an observer from the *outside* does not *and* cannot see. It is important to have both the outer *and* the inner perceptions of what is happening in the treatment of an illness. This is important both in *our* life *and* in our patients' lives. *One without the other is not complete.* As we watch a small child or animal look at and play with its reflection in a mirror, we begin to get a glimpse of how we, as evolving conscious beings, can become acquainted with and get to know ourselves as we manifest in this reality. At this stage of my life, I look in the mirror and wonder who that "old" woman is, because, *internally,* I do *not* feel like what I *look* like in the mirror! Yet I know that *both* the inner and the outer are real. Because I am such a proponent of "aging into health," what *I* see in the mirror never really bothers me. I just see someone who is *living* her life and is in the process of what I call aging into health!

9

The Garden

Essential to our house of Living Medicine is our front and back yards, the garden and even the air that encircles our home. Just like what we allow *into* our home greatly impacts us, we need to recognize that what we allow into the areas *surrounding* our dwelling place can likewise impact us. The front yard of our house of Living Medicine is what we *consciously* present to the world. It is the focus of our life which the rest of the world sees, such as where we put our lights and Christmas decorations and the face we present to the world. Our backyard represents our *unconscious* mind and our unconscious being, where life goes on in ways that the rest of the world does *not* see or need to see, unless we *choose* to let them see it.

As physicians, part of our job is recognizing that a patient who comes into our office initially presents us with their *front* yard...what they *want* us to see *or* what they have created in the way of a façade for the world to see. That is fine, because it gives us a sense of who they either *think* they are OR who they want *other people* to think they are. If we as physicians truly want to work with healing the underlying *causes* of disease, instead of just treating the symptoms, we need to be able to step into that person's *back*yard and see what has been stored there. In the *back*yard is where we will find *what* even *our patients may not want to see*, much less show off, which could be the basis of the *cause* of the disease that has been created. Frequently, a patient will come into my office complaining of a sore throat or a bad shoulder. If all I do is give them an antibiotic or a prescription for pain medicine, I have done something with their *front* yard in order to make it look and feel better. If we get into their *back*yard, we may find that the sore throat is there because this person has been trying to say something that they have not been able to say. They may have been "swallowing words" that they were unable to express, *or* they may have been screaming for attention for a long time and not getting any response or felt *truly* heard. **Whatever the core issues are that have been stored in our patients' *back*yards need to be revealed, acknowledged and worked with before *true* healing can happen.** If a patient presents with a sore shoulder, what we may find in their *back*yard is that they have been "shouldering" too much responsibility for their household, *or* they may be shouldering somebody else's cares. They could also be carrying a purse that is too heavy *or* doing some physical activities that need to be changed so as not to cause pain.

Every house of Living Medicine has some sort of a backdoor. The tents in which we lived when I was a child in the jungles of India had a backflap. Every house that I have ever lived in has had a backdoor. The purpose for the backdoor, among other things, is that it gives us a way we can come and go without being noticed. If left improperly closed, uninvited guests might enter my home. These can be actual persons, pets, concepts, emotions, spiritual ideologies or, as often happens, disease processes. Sometimes, we do not know these things are there. When we discover them, however, we can either choose to ignore their presence *or* allow them to settle in. Two very different examples follow, one trivial in nature and one very serious.

One night, after I had spent three sleepless nights tossing and turning because of certain issues and problems that were manifesting in my life at the time, I went to bed at ten o'clock. I dropped into a deep sleep, then was suddenly awakened at midnight by a big thump. Our indoor/outdoor cat had jumped on my bed and began padding his way across it. I, of course, jumped out of bed, talked to him and tried to get him to leave, yet he would not. Instead, he jumped down off the bed and climbed underneath my rocking chair, which has a skirt around the bottom, and stayed there. I tried coaxing him out and pushing him from behind, yet he would not budge. When I tried to reach in and pull him out, he hissed at me. This scenario went on for about an hour. I finally decided to get back into bed and try to get some sleep, since he was not about to move. I had just dozed off when he jumped back up on my bed. This time, I got out of bed and grabbed him. I told him he was symbolic of my fears and anxieties, then tossed him out the backdoor and locked it. In that moment, I realized that our huge, smart tomcat had figured out how to get in the backdoor that I had forgotten to lock earlier in the evening!

In the second example, the importance of the backdoor became very clear to me when I was working with a friend. As a counselor and massage therapist, she had spent her life taking good care of her body, as well as taking care of her friends and relatives. She was also totally devoted to her environment, including her garden and her pets. She adored her family, her parents, her siblings and her children. She grew up on health foods, understood how to use herbs and essential oils, had used castor oil packs, done biofeedback, knew the importance of meditation and prayer and had used *all* of this knowledge in her life. She was a person who had kept diaries and journals ever since she was a young girl. When she discovered a lump in her breast, she used a castor oil pack on it. The lump went away for a while. When it came back, she added some visualization and dietary changes, which helped. She continued caring for herself in a healthy, loving way. When the lump did *not* respond, she increased her visualization and *worked harder* on trying to get rid of the lump. She continued to love her body in every way she knew how. Despite all her efforts, however, the lump grew. She then began to feel guilty, thinking there must be something that she had or had not done to create this lump. Because of her feelings of not wanting to disrupt her family's situation or the life that she had so carefully constructed, she continued to carry this burden *all by herself*. She finally realized that she needed help and spoke to her family and a physician about her condition. She then began the process of moving into the medical system to get the lump removed, which she did, then followed up with chemotherapy. We had many in-depth conversations about what was *really* going on. She said she felt like the lump was symbolic of her having allowed her teenage son to bring his rowdy, disruptive friends in through her "backdoor." True to her nature, though, she took care of her son's friends, making sure they had food and water, places to sleep and anything else they thought they needed, because she loved her son. Now, however, these "friends" had taken over her house and were in the process of destroying it. She said she felt that, although she had loved and cared for her breasts like she had cared for her home, she now realized she had allowed the rowdy teenagers to destroy *her* dwelling place. It was hard for her to say: "They have to get out. I must get rid of something that I have created *both* within my own *home* and now within my own *body*. I've created this lump, because I've allowed cells that weren't welcome in my body to grow and displace the healthy cells. They've left their toxic waste and debris everywhere, and they have no respect for me and my house. It's time for them to go." She then visualized the surgeon and the surgery as the sheriff coming in and evicting these young people. After they were gone, the chemotherapy represented the clean-up team that came in to clean up the mess the teenagers had left behind. But for *true* healing to happen, she had to reestablish who owned the house, who was going to take care of it and who was truly responsible for it. She became Athena, the warrior princess, who was able to get rid of an invading army. She stepped into the role of "tough love." To allow life to flow well in her home once more, she had to be discerning as to who and what she was going to have *stay,* and who and what she was going to have *go,* so that she could get on with her, which is what she did.

There are times in our lives when living our life requires a battle. There are times when we need to prune our trees or weed our garden. There are times when a tooth needs to be pulled or an abscess needs to be drained. There are times when an antibiotic is *absolutely* essential in order for life to go on. We may have a backyard where a great deal of fun, joy and play are expressed. We may have a beautiful garden growing in our backyard, which demonstrates a beautiful soul and Spirit. However, this beauty will only manifest in a *lasting* way when we also choose to take care of the larger garden of Mother Earth.

We are both very much aware about the lack of concern for renewable fuels in our world. The idea that we can keep draining oil from the earth and that there is an *endless* supply is totally irresponsible and very dangerous. *Oil is the earth's lifeblood.* As physicians, we are very aware of the importance of caring for our physical bodies. We really need to treat them with loving respect. By the same token, we need to look at Mother Earth as a Living Body that has a *limited supply of energy.* Just as it is within our own bodies, **if we exhaust our energy supply, we can no longer function**. If we exhaust the energy supply that is available to us from Mother Earth, we will destroy Her.

In 2000, I started driving a Honda Insight, one of the first hybrid cars. Because they start with gas and then run on electricity, they do not need to plug in or attach to electrical outlets. These hybrid cars are now readily available, as well as other vehicles that use renewable fuel, in addition to the *fully*-electric car. By choosing a car like this, we are doing a better job in caring for Mother Earth. This is one way we can care for our planet's resources, as well as teach our children, grandchildren and great-grandchildren to be responsible stewards of these resources.

I have a friend who says: "It's time we stopped digging in the ground for oil in the Middle East and begin to dig for water for the people in Africa." *Water is more precious than oil, and the continent of Africa is dying of thirst.* Water *itself* does not pollute! We would serve our world better if we changed our focus from *dead* fossil fuels to water, which is in endless supply and is a *living* resource. *We cannot live without water—we* can *live without oil.*

We consider ourselves smart people. Yet, we do these really foolish things that not only jeopardize *our* health, they also jeopardize the health of future generations. It is time we stop polluting our world and begin to take care of our beautiful Mother Earth in earnest. Our

Native American brothers and sisters know how important it is to do this. They know that when a plant is cut, Mother Earth needs to be thanked for giving us that plant. They thank Her also for the fish from the streams and for the animals from the woods. They use *everything* that they take from Mother Earth, wasting nothing, allowing Her to easily renew Her supply. *We are totally dependent on Mother Earth. She is very accommodating to us, even though we continue to take Her for granted and cause Her great suffering.* I believe, metaphorically, that we are causing Mother Earth to have osteoporosis by continually removing Her minerals, coal and other substances that cannot be replaced. *We* all *need to learn to live in harmony with* all *of Mother Nature and be willing to learn the lessons that She so generously provides for us* and *our patients.*

In earlier cultures, when the *feminine* nature of our humanness was respected and predominant, we had an agrarian culture with no walls. People learned to live together, and they came and went with ease. Fights or disagreements were dealt with out in the open. When the *masculine* nature of our being became dominant, we created *walls* to keep people out. It became "us against them." We had to protect what was ours, and anything outside of the wall became an enemy. This practice ultimately resulted in the Dark Ages, where corruption and destruction happened *within* the walls. The *whole* growth cycle imploded upon itself. We are now moving into a new era where *the feminine is re-emerging* and being respected for her nurturing nature. A good example of this is the day the Berlin Wall came down. It was one of the happiest days of my life. There was *global* excitement and jubilation. It saddens me to see that walls are being recreated in many places; not *that all walls are bad.* There are times when walls are necessary. It is what walls are *used for* and *our reason for creating them* that needs to be recognized. For example, walls can create a contained area where beauty, love and nature come together in a garden to create a sacred space. My little meditation garden, encompassed within a low wall, represents one way in which I can access aspects of my being that otherwise I might not be able to access. This is especially true on the *unconscious* level. It is a riot of color, with very little structure, because I get very excited when a *volunteer* plant comes up. I even have some weeds that I consider very beautiful! I have trouble pulling them out, although sometimes they need to be removed so that the *other* plants have a chance to really grow and thrive. My garden is truly a way of expressing my own creative abilities, and it reflects who I am. It also allows me to observe Life in the process of growing and becoming *new* life, which gives me hope and joy. Its wall gives my climbing plants an opportunity to grow and thrive, including those that show up in my garden as volunteers. The following story is a great illustration of this idea.

About twenty years ago, I noticed a little sprout coming up in my garden. I did not know what it was. Because it was pretty, I just watched it grow. As it continued to grow, it became a tree with feathery leaves just outside of my library window. It is a very pleasant tree, and I have become very fond of it. Through the years, nobody seemed to know what this tree was, until a friend of mine said: "That's a silk oak." I had never heard of a silk oak and thought: "Well, at least I have a name for it now." When I went to India in February 2005, I saw this same kind of tree growing all over the part of India where I grew up! I asked my friend (Pavitra) about this tree, and she immediately replied that it was a silk oak. When I returned home, I searched the internet to find out more about silk oaks, because I had never seen one in the Phoenix area. I found out that silk oaks *do* grow in southern Arizona! Since it is growing right against the wall of my house, my daughter (Helene) became concerned that its roots would damage the foundation of my home. What I discovered was that the roots of the silk oak go very deep and can be planted next to a house *without* affecting the foundation in any way. The amazing thing to me is that for some reason, the Powers That Be allowed the seed of this tree to be planted in *my* little meditation garden. How that happened, I will never know. I just marvel that it connected me to my birthplace, to the very soil of the countryside where I grew up. A little hummingbird also loves to sit on one of the branches of this tree. As I write these words, I see it sitting there. The bird will stay there for up to an hour at a time, just looking around and being beautiful in my little silk oak. To me, this silk oak tree represents the wonderful connection that we have with Mother Earth and the amazing way She will respond to us as we become aware of Her and She becomes aware of us. What is it in my *unconscious* that called out to the silk oak seed the message that having this little tree grow in my garden would mean so much to me? I truly believe *we are all connected and that our needs are known and will always be taken care of.*

Some of the plants in my garden have been started from seed in a pot, like my little papaya plant. Its little pot provides the protective "walls" it needs to get a strong start in the world. It is growing very well and, at some point in time, when its roots have stretched out far enough, I will take it out of the little pot and put it in the ground so it can continue to grow. If I do not remove those "walls" when my little papaya plant no longer needs them, it will become rootbound in the pot. Ultimately, its growth would be restricted, and it would probably die. So when I put it in the ground and properly fertilize and care for it, it will grow into a tall papaya tree. As it produces fruit and seed, it will perpetuate the life of the little papaya plant.

Our lives can be very much like this little papaya plant, in that *we* start out needing a "protected space" in which to grow and be nurtured. Then there comes a time when we are asked to reach beyond that protective space and stretch our roots farther so we can continue to grow, so that life can go on. Just like the pot for my little papaya plant represents walls that are sometimes needed for the plant to take root and grow, *children* also need to grow within the walls of a home, until they are strong enough to move out. Their thoughts and emotions likewise need to have a safe space in which to grow and become strong. Then they can learn to recognize *their* thoughts and emotions for what they are and allow them to be part of *their* garden. We *all* need some boundaries, so we can identify *our own* individuality and learn who *we* really are. Our personality develops and can grow safely within these boundaries. *We cannot live our whole life behind walls.*

There comes a time when, just as the little papaya plant needs to be taken out of *its* pot, *we* must step outside of *our* garden wall and meet the world. *Until then*, however, our homes and classrooms should be *safe* places where we can grow and become strong enough to step out into the world with confidence and assurance.

Friendships are like the plants that grow in our garden. They *all require care*, even the weeds and the "volunteers" that arrive uninvited. *Each one* can enrich our lives in *some* way, *if* we can allow and appreciate each one's *unique* contribution. This principle was demonstrated to me recently when I was talking to someone who was really upset about the breaking up of a relationship that she had thought of as a lifelong friendship. She said she was just not interested in "superficial" friendships, since in her words: "they're a waste of time and energy." We talked a long time about this and about how *some casual relationships can* truly *change people's lives*, even if we do not recognize that fact in the moment. Just as the daisy has *shallow* roots and the oak has *deep* ones, *both* have their special place in this world of ours and are important. The daisy has as much right to live in this world and bring beauty, despite its "superficial" roots, as does the oak with its deep, deep roots.

Every house of Living Medicine has its own compost area, whether it is a dedicated compost pit or just scattered table scraps. Whether we are *consciously* aware of it or not, it is where organic material is disposed of, so that it can decompose and become *living* substance once again. On a *physical* level, it is the *actual* organic materials that we throw away. On a *mental* level, it can be the thoughts and concepts that no longer serve us and are ready to be transformed. On the *emotional* level, it can represent the feelings we are now ready to release, so that they can be resolved and find their rightful place within our ever-growing soul. On a *spiritual* level, if there are ideologies and theologies that no longer serve us, we can let them go into the compost pit so that they can emerge as something that is truly life-*giving* and healthy. *Out of the compost pit,* new *life can grow.* It is *not* necessary to go to the compost pit, pick up every banana peel or eggshell to look at and dissect. Mother Nature understands and knows the importance of taking the materials that we return to her physically, mentally, emotionally and spiritually. She can recycle and reuse these materials in such a way that Life becomes an ongoing, continuous *living* cycle. Jesus said it this way (italics are mine): "My Father is a gardener. Every *barren* branch of mine He cuts away, and every *fruiting* branch He cleans to make it more fruitful still. *This is my Father's glory, that you bear fruit and plenty*" (John 15:1-3).

This idea was poignantly demonstrated to me during the last week of September 2001 when I happened to turn on my television and saw the movie *To Sir, With Love II,* the 1997 sequel to the 1967 film. In this movie, Sidney Poitier returns from London and comes into a rough and wild high school in the slums of Chicago. When he enters the classroom the first day, there is fighting and general chaos. He must break up at least one of the fights in order to get any attention at all. One of the first things he does with the children in this classroom is to ask them a simple question, requiring each of them to answer it one at a time: "Who are you?" As they replied with cocky answers about who *they* thought they were, the other children responded to their answers in derogatory ways, since *they* saw their classmates differently than those students saw themselves. It took time, though gradually these students began to really look at themselves and see who they *really* were. This was quite different from the way they had seen themselves *initially*, including the image they had portrayed to others. *Each one of them had believed themselves to be losers.* They had felt that there was no way out of the situation in which they found themselves, except by fighting and rebelling. As they began to look *within*, however, they found talents and abilities they could access that they had not known they had. The students came to realize that they could really *like* themselves. By the time they graduated, many no longer saw themselves as losers. Instead, *they began to see themselves as genuine people who could contribute to society*...and they were *forever* changed. In this example, the classroom was like the compost pit when Sidney Poitier came into it, and the children certainly saw themselves as compost. Over time, though, with a great deal of tender nurturing, the "Master Gardener" (Poitier) transformed that compost pit into a beautiful garden.

In our discussion together about this story, Dr. Ann pointed out that, in a way, Sidney Poitier had actually followed Stephen Covey's "success formula" with his students: if you "sow a thought, [you] reap an action; [if you] sow an action, [you] reap a habit; [if you] sow a habit, [you] reap a character; [if you] sow a character, [you] reap a destiny."[220] Because the teacher (Poitier) *was* masterful in the way he tended his "garden" (his classroom), his students lives *were* changed forever, because he showed them the way to fulfill their individual destinies (or life purposes). Dr. Ann then shared with me how another film (*Johnny Lingo*), the storyline of which was originally written and published as a short story set in a Polynesian culture[221] and demonstrated *this same principle*, was introduced to her by one of her college professors in 1969 and forever changed *her* life in a similarly profound way. I encourage you to see the original film[222] or its expanded version[223] on Netflix.

I live by the concept that there must be *some* way in which I can learn to love myself, so that I can be a *living example* of the following principle: **in *every* moment of *every* day, as physicians *and* patients, we have the opportunity to *choose* whether we are going to be losers or winners.** The struggle is *not* about winning a war against people on the *outside*. Rather, it is about resolving the struggle that goes on in every moment *within* ourselves. Just like the little papaya plant, we have come to a point now in our lives where we need to take ourselves out of the restraining confines of the *self-created* pot in which we have been growing, feeling like a loser. We must *now* plant ourselves in Mother Earth in such a way that we can extend our

---

[220] Covey, Stephen. The 7 Habits of Highly Successful People, 1989.

[221] McGerr, Patricia. "Johnny Lingo and the Eight-Cow Wife" in Woman's Day Magazine, 1965.

[222] m.imdb.com>JohnnyLingo(1969).

[223] https://flixlist.co>TheLegendofJohnnyLingo-2003.

roots into the world around us. Then we can grow into the reality of who we *truly* are, producing the fruit that only *we* can produce. This is best achieved from full, expanded, healthy living. **How we *each* live our individual lives matters!** *Each* **of us creates the world we individually live in**—perhaps not the circumstances, though how we *respond to* what happens to us in those circumstances is what *truly* matters. This is the garden (world) we are leaving to our children. How *we* blossom and bloom in *our* Living Medicine garden is our gift to them and to the world.

We are all aware that plants convert carbon dioxide into oxygen, which is essential for *our* very existence on this planet. However, *research is now showing that plants, by* their *very existence, can help us emotionally and spiritually, as well as physically.* There are research projects[224] that have taken a small plant into nursing homes, where the elderly are frequently depressed and unable to care for *themselves* OR respond to anyone or anything *outside* of themselves. If these folks are given a plant to take care of, so they can nurture it and see it grow, many times their life takes on new meaning. A pet can also be very useful therapy in this setting.[225] **If we surround ourselves with *living* things, our life is enriched abundantly.** Research that supports this principle in an amazing and profound way was done by Bill Thomas, MD and his wife (Jude Meyers-Thomas), cofounders of The Eden Alternative®.[226] It was conducted at the Chase Memorial Nursing Home in New Berlin, New York in the early 1990's over a two-year period. A delightful article about this study and how The Eden Alternative® came to be is well worth reading.[227,228] *In a nutshell*: Dr. Thomas, a Harvard-trained physician and out-of-the-box thinker,

---

[224] https://www.sciencedaily.com/releases/2009/02/090226134813.htm.

[225] https://www.ncbi.nlm.nih.gov>pmc4248608.

[226] Thomas, William H., MD. Life Worth Living: How Someone You Love Can Still Enjoy Life in a Nursing Home, 1996.

[227] www.changingaging.org>blog>can>life>in>a>nursing>home>be>made>uplifting> and>purposeful (reprinted from the book below).

[228] Gawande, Atul, MD. Being Mortal: Medicine and What Matters in the End, 2014 and 2017.

became Chase's medical director after working in the ER for many years, primarily because he wanted a "day job" so he could stop working nights. He tried many different *conventional* medicine therapies with the residents for a period of time, "none of which really worked." After purchasing land and beginning to farm it, he saw that "what was missing [in the nursing home] was Life itself." He soon thereafter correctly diagnosed the "problem" that *all* the residents had in common: "the Three Plagues—boredom, loneliness and helplessness." Within two years, he discovered that the solutions to those "plagues" were spontaneity, companionship and a chance to feel needed by taking care of another "being" (green plants in *every* room, vegetable and flower gardens instead of lawn. and a *myriad* of different animals— nearly 200 in all!). *He changed everything at once,* creating a form of "shock therapy," where daily life at Chase went from "total pandemonium" to "glorious chaos" within a few months. He said he chose to make the transition in this way to purposefully disrupt the "inertia of [the nursing home] culture…[where] institutional routines and safety [were] greater priorities than living a good life." His definition of a good life? "Maximum independence." He compared his residents' progress over the two years to a traditional nursing home (the "control" group in the study). The outcome? His residents' number of prescription medications fell to one-half of the number of Rx's prescribed in the control group, especially psychotropic Rx's for agitation. In addition, drug costs at Chase were thirty-eight percent of the control group's medication costs, and deaths at Chase were fifteen percent less than in the control group. Dr. Thomas said: "It's not so much about the decrease in the death rate [as it is about] the fundamental human need for a reason to live"—a person's ideal or life purpose, in my view, which is why I *always* ask patients this question when they consult with me. "The residents began to wake up and come to life…the lights turned back on in people's eyes." Who knew that plants and pets could create such a change! As a result of this amazing research and one pioneering physician's commitment to make a difference, The

Eden Alternative® is being adopted in many other communities, both nationally and internationally.[229]

In the Bible (Deuteronomy 30:19), it says (italics are mine): "I have set before you life and death, blessing and cursing, therefore *choose life* that both thou and thy seed may live." *Every moment of every day we are making choices.* Our Living Medicine garden must, by its very nature, include the world *outside* of any walls, so that *the whole earth becomes our garden*. It becomes *our* Garden of Eden when we begin to think of the earth as *our* responsibility and our involvement in Life itself as being part of what is going on in it. Then we can, and *will*, take responsibility for caring and loving Mother Earth. It will require a level of understanding that *we can no longer pollute our streams and our oceans with our refuse* to the point that we are killing the water creatures. **Matter does *not* disappear**, based on the Law of Conservation of Mass.[230] **It can only be changed from one form to another**, as the *female* mathematician and physicist Èmilie du Châtelet was the *first* to conclude in 1740 also about energy.[231] When the pollutants we discard into our streams are transformed into toxic materials that injure water creatures, we are causing *severe harm* to the ENTIRE ecosystem, including ourselves. The *soil* in which our plants grow is also no longer nourishing when we put toxic materials in it that Mother Earth cannot transform into healthy substances. I am constantly amazed at the way in which Mother Nature has and does transform our pollutants. However, *there comes a tipping point where She can no longer tolerate this abuse. We need to accept responsibility and*

---

[229] www.edenalt.org.

[230] Lavoisier, Antoine. "Matter is neither created nor destroyed" (the Law of Conservation of Mass),1785; Mayer, Julius R. "Energy is neither created nor destroyed" (the Law of Conservation of Energy, now called the First Law of Thermodynamics), 1742; and Einstein, Albert. Merged these two laws after his discovery of the equation $E=mc^2$ into the Law of Conservation of Mass-Energy: "The total amount of mass and energy in the universe is constant," 1907) www.chemteam. info>thermochem>Law-of-Conservation-of-Mass-Energy.

[231] du Châtelet, Èmilie. The first to propose, test and publish The Law of Conservation of Energy in 1740 www.en.m.wikipedia.org>Conservation_of_Energy and www. en.m.wikipedia.org>Èmilie_du_Châtelet.

help Her with Her healing. The 2020 coronavirus pandemic is a perfect example of this problem. As a result of it, a near-global shutdown of our world as we have known it has been required. Consequently, Mother Earth is responding to what *we* have done to Her by transforming the *lack* of pollutants into *clean* air, since *we* have failed in our responsibility to keep the air that we breathe clean. Likewise, in our bodies, if we continually pollute them, there also comes a tipping point where natural and living forces can no longer heal us, and we die. Our house of Living Medicine must be built on *living* earth. It must have *living* water available to it, *living* air surrounding it and *living* plants embracing it. *Living* animals must also dwell in it, as well as *living* birds surrounding it, with their songs and beauty gladdening the heart of our home. Even *living* insects must be present to supply food for the birds. As humans, for us to continue to live on Mother Earth, we must keep Her alive, treat Her with respect, love Her and stop destroying the very Essence of who and what She is.

10

The Back Porch

When we step out of our backdoor, we step onto the back porch. Chairs and places to sit are arranged there, especially so we can see what goes on in our backyard and also watch the sunset.

Watching sunsets has been very important in my life. In Arizona we have some of the most spectacular sunsets in the world. I mentioned this to some friends one day. Their collective response was basically: "But that is when the evening news comes on." So, in keeping up with "the news," they were missing the grand color and light show of Life. The evening news tells us about things that have happened during that day. It does *not* tell us about the precious moments that have filled our day, such as the sunset itself. *If you don't look, you can't see, and you can miss the grandeur of Life itself.* Jesus said: "He who has eyes to see, let him see and ears to hear, let him hear" (Mark 4:9-12).

One of my most important memories related to watching a sunset occurred as a teenager in India, while sitting in the swing on our back porch with my Aunt Belle. It was a clear early evening in the foothills of the Himalayan Mountains, and we were watching a glorious sunset. Aunt Belle asked me if I knew what a sunset was. When I said no, she told me that it was a gift from God...that with each sunset, God opened a window into heaven and let us have a view of what heaven is like. I accepted and loved Aunt Belle's view of a sunset.

As I grew into adulthood, my view of heaven expanded. I was a mother with children of my own before I finally figured out *my* concept of heaven. I became aware that when Jesus said: "the kingdom of heaven is within you" (Luke 17:21), He probably meant that we were creating our heaven here on earth, day by day. Our thoughts, our emotions and the things that we do create the world we live in. We can put our attention on the things around us that bring light and joy into the world (like a sunset), or we can attend to what causes pain and hardship. *It is our choice.* I have had glimpses of heaven in the face of a newborn baby, in the faces of patients when they awaken to the reality that the Physician Within them is *truly* a part of themselves, while sitting at a table surrounded by my children and grandchildren and even while kissing a "boo-boo" when my children hurt their knees. I have seen heaven in the face of the housemother Pavitra Masih in India, as she cared for the children of leper parents. I have seen it in the faces of Afghani women when they learn something new about their own bodies and about birthing babies. The windows of heaven for *me* were thrown wide open in 2007 when my daughter (Analea) died in my bed, with the whole family present, surrounding her with love. *Every new day, in one way or another, offers me opportunities to create my heavenly reality on earth.* Now, as I watch sunsets, I am constantly reminded that it is part of my mission to attend to and recognize the beauty of each one.

We as humans are meant to be social beings, regardless of our life circumstances. We need each other. Some of us have been fortunate enough to have created community within a healthy family structure, large or small. Others of us have created a more solitary life, within a family or social community of choice. *No matter what kind of social community we have created, we still need each other.* Even a monk living a solitary life in a cave in the Himalayas still has a community that brings them food. It is now a well-established scientific fact that babies can die if they are not properly touched as newborns, as previously discussed in chapter three. As we were writing this paragraph, the following article[232] appeared in the news (bold is mine):

---

[232] Trinko, Katrina. Opinion columnist. USA Today. May 3, 2018.

Gen Z is the Loneliest Generation, and It's Not Just Because of Social Media

The loneliness of Generation Z reflects not just rising social media use but a broader decline in interactions with neighbors, co-workers and church friends.

At a time when we're supposedly more connected than ever, there are an awful lot of lonely people.

"Nearly half of Americans report sometimes or always feeling alone or left out, according to a new survey from health company Cigna (https:// www.multivu.com/players/English/8294451-cigna-us-loneliness-survey/)." **One out of five Americans has no person they can talk to.**

And the loneliest generation? (https://www. cigna.com/assets/docs/newsroom/loneliness-survey-2018-full-report.pdf). That would be **Generation Z**, *defined in this survey as those* **18 to 22**. *Their average loneliness score is nearly 10 points higher than* **the least lonely generation—the Greatest Generation, those 72 and older.**

While it's tempting to blame Gen Z's reliance on smartphones and social media, the data don't bear that out: that survey didn't find a significant difference in loneliness levels between those who used social media often or infrequently.

Given the worrying consequences, **the loneliness of Gen Z —and other generations— should be taken seriously.** *In fact, Cigna, citing a 2010* Brigham Young University study (https://journals.sagepub.com/doi/abs/10.1177/1745691614568352), *says* **"loneliness has the same impact on mortality as smoking 15 cigarettes a day, making it even more dangerous than obesity."**

One initiative to encourage Gen Z should be #WalkUpNotOut (https://www.cnn.com/2018/03/14/us/ryan-petty-walk-up-walk-out-stoneman-douglas-shooting-trnd/index.html), *a movement that urged high school students to reach out to students perceived as socially isolated after the tragic high school shooting in Parkland, Fla. Regardless of your position on gun control, it can only help to have students focus on being kind and welcoming to each other, particularly when the pervasiveness of social media has made it increasingly easy to bully, both on and off campuses.*

Plus, this encourages face-to-face interaction— *and the Cigna survey found* **a huge difference in average loneliness scores between those who had** *daily* **meaningful in-person encounters and those who didn't.** *(Astonishingly, one of five Americans surveyed reported having such encounters less frequently than once a week.)*

It's also important for Gen Z—and other Americans—to take "social capital" seriously. Thanks to the erosion of neighborhood communities, the fracturing of many families and the decline in church attendance, there are fewer and fewer opportunities for finding new friends or developing meaningful relationships. And that puts even more pressure on students. **Imagine being unhappy at school and having no other community to turn to.**

According to a 2017 report prepared for Sen. Mike Lee, R-Utah, several factors show the <u>decline in our interaction with each other</u> (<u>https://www.lee.senate.gov/public/_cache/files/b5f-224ce-98f7-40f6-a814-8602696714d8/what-we-do-together.pdf</u>):

- *Monthly **church attendance** fell from the early 1970's.*
- *In 1974, a third of Americans **spent time socially with their neighbors** several times a week. Now, only 19% do.*
- *We're also spending less time **schmoozing with our co-workers**, going from an average of 2.5 hours a week in the mid-1970's to just under an hour in 2012.*
- ***Families are also becoming smaller,** and the percentage of children raised by a single parent or no parent has doubled, from 15% to 31%.*

*Given these declining numbers, it makes sense that **more Americans are falling through the cracks, losing ways to get to know other people**.*

And if Gen Z is using phones instead of in-person interactions, that could be contributing to these young adults' loneliness. In an <u>Atlantic</u> article last year, psychology professor Jean Twenge highlighted how teens were less interested in driving and getting out of the house than past generations.

Describing one unnamed 13-year-old, Twenge wrote: "She spent much of her summer keeping up with friends, but nearly <u>all of it was over text or Snapchat (https://www.theatlantic.com/ magazine/archive/2017/09/has-the-smart-phone-destroyed-a-generation/534198/).</u> **'I've been on my phone more than I've been with actual people,'** *she said, 'My bed has, like, an imprint of my body,'"*

That's not healthy—and if these are the habits Gen Z is developing in these crucial years, it doesn't bode well for this generation becoming less lonely in the future.

The American writer Flannery O'Connor, a Catholic, was fond of a prayer that included these lines, "Raphael, lead us toward those we are waiting for, those who are waiting for us: Raphael, Angel of happy meeting, lead us by the hand toward those we are looking for."

You don't need to be religious to realize that **we both need—and are needed by—others**, *and that our own lives grow in meaning through many of our interactions with others.*

It's easy to toss out opinions on Facebook or on bumper stickers, but at the end of the day, one of the most powerful things many of us may do to change the world could be our "hello" to someone, our reaching out to that person who seems in danger of being on the fringe, making eye contact and sharing a smile with a homeless person, even if we don't have change. **Let's look up from our phones a little more often—and start acknowledging the people right in front of us.**

Let us take this entire article to heart, especially the admonitions in the last paragraph. As Dr. Ann said to me when she gave me this article to read: "We *have* to include this! It reminds me so much of a principle I learned from Stephen Covey[233] a long time ago (italics are ours): **'Things which matter most must *never* be at the mercy of things which matter least.'**" I couldn't agree more. No doubt "sheltering in place" during the 2020 coronavirus pandemic has contributed somewhat to alleviating the loneliness this article points out, though we do not believe that it has *corrected* it. However, it has given parents an opportunity to become re-acquainted with their children *and* each other! This is a perfect example of how the Universe takes what we have messed up and attempts to fix it.

I have a wonderful friend who is an old lady like I am. She is a perfect example of Living Medicine in action with respect to the importance of creating community to stay healthy and alive. Her husband died a few years ago, and she has continued to live a life of outreach and service. I was talking to her recently, and she told me about a young man from Egypt that she was working with who spoke no English, though he had two PhD's in different subjects. *With all his ability and knowledge, he had no social community.* He was finding himself isolated, lonely and depressed. She offered to go with him to

---

[233] Covey, Stephen. The 7 Habits of Highly Successful People, 1989.

court, so that he could get some of his identity papers clarified. This one "random act of kindness"[234] and caring *made all the difference* in the world for him at that time. She is dignified in her appearance and presentation and was like a ray of hope for him at a crucial time in his life. My friend is helping him not only learn English, they are also creating a social community *together*. In so doing, he has been able to find himself again, and she now also has social community in *her* life. She is truly a person who creates community wherever she goes.

The concepts of Living Medicine have become more and more important in the field of medicine as *conventional* **practice moves deeper and deeper into the war against diseases.** The literature that physicians continually receive focuses on "pay for performance" activity in their practices and in the hospitals where they practice. Insurance companies have established certain criteria and parameters that need to be maintained for specific diseases (such as hypertension) in which the "normal" blood pressure must be held at 130/80 mm Hg. In diabetes, the blood sugar needs to fall below 100 mg/dL to be considered "normal." With cholesterol, the total amount must be kept below 200 mg/dL, while the HDL and LDL must be kept within very specific limits to be considered "normal." *Physicians are now being told that* only *when they can keep at least a certain number of their patients at these required levels can they expect their income to increase.* Hospitals are being told what medications they need to give a patient the moment that person enters the emergency room with a cardiac episode. *If the hospital follows that regimen precisely, it will receive* higher *reimbursement.* Unfortunately, these requirements do not take into consideration the *patients* who do very, very poorly on certain medications prescribed to keep their blood sugar, blood pressure or cholesterol down. **The** *mandated* **criteria and parameters do** *not* **take into consideration** *individual* **variants** which, of course, are part of treating a patient as an *individual.* **In Living Medicine, we can look at such mandates and change that which**

---

[234] Conari Press (editors). Random Acts of Kindness, 2002 and Random Acts of Kindness Then & Now, 2013 (20th Anniversary ed.).

needs to be changed *without* penalizing physicians' reimbursements.

Drug companies have pushed hard to make certain drugs mandatory *for the treatment of certain diseases.* Insurance companies' "formularies" do not give credence to alternative therapeutic medicines. They also refuse to pay for "experimental" treatments (e.g. biofeedback, exercise, diet and laughter). Despite a myriad of research showing the effectiveness of these therapies, they still claim they are not "evidence-based." Their entire focus is on prescription medications and *conventional* therapeutic interventions. *Many of these medications and interventions have iatrogenic consequences* (side effects caused by a medication or therapy prescribed by a physician), which then require another medication or intervention to correct *that* problem. There is no end to the problems constantly being created if *conventional* medicine continues to travel down this road. *Only when we take a* life-giving *approach to health and focus on what it takes for* true *healing to happen, will we be able to move off of the dark and frightening path on which many physicians now find themselves.*

For the most part, ***conventional* medicine (in all its forms) is so busy trying to prevent death that it is killing Life.** *No wonder physician burnout has become so common,* even among its best and most well-trained physicians. To address this problem *effectively,* I believe that physicians who are still predominantly practicing in a *conventional* manner must ***first* be open to the possibility of a paradigm shift in** their **thinking.** I also agree with Stephen Covey[235] who said: "the more aware we are of our basic paradigms...or assumptions, and the extent to which we have been influenced by our experience, the more we can take responsibility for those paradigms...[and then] examine them, test them against reality, listen to others and be open to their perceptions, thereby [gaining] a larger picture and a far more objective view." Applying this principle to medicine, Covey goes on to say (bold, italics and capitals are mine): "The more people are into 'quick fix' and focus on...*acute* problems and pain, the more that

---

[235] Covey, Stephen. The 7 Habits of Highly Effective People, 1989.

very approach contributes to the underlying *chronic* condition....But the underlying chronic condition remains and, eventually, new acute symptoms will appear. ***The way we see the problem IS the problem.***" We as physicians will never see what we are *unwilling* to see, and physician burnout is only *one* of the results of that kind of thinking.

Another kind of thinking that can result in physician burnout is *perfectionism,* as Natasha Frost describes:[236] "In 1950, the German psychoanalyst Karen Horney described perfectionists as being terrorized by the 'tyranny of the should'—that they felt they 'should' be any number of contradictory ideals, able to solve any problem, complete impossible tasks and so on....In the decades since then, perfectionism has been found to be closely *correlated* personally *with mental health issues* (depression, anxiety, eating disorders). Professionally, it *can lead to burnout and stress*....On the other hand, perfectionists have been found to be more motivated and conscientious than their nonperfectionistic peers, both highly desirable traits in the [workplace].... Forthcoming research from Phillips University of Marburg in Germany, however, suggests that there is a 'null' relationship between perfectionism and performance, meaning it is *not a trait that is positive or negative*....A 2018 analysis from British researchers [ ] investigated more than 40,000 college students' answers to a 'perfectionism scale' questionnaire, compiled between 1986 and 2015. The results were clear: *young people are far more likely to be perfectionists than their predecessors.* Recent college students, whether millennials [anyone born between 1981 and 1996] or Generation Z [anyone born between 1997 and 2012],[237] perceive others as expecting more from them while simultaneously having higher expectations of themselves and those around them."

While we *do* need physicians who are motivated and conscientious, I think that physician burnout and stress is much too high a price to pay for those traits. I have always said (and lived by) the philosophy

---

[236] Frost, Natasha. https://worklife/article/20200715-why-no-one-wants-to-work-with-a-perfectionist.

[237] Dimock, Michael. www.pewresearch.org>defining-generations (January 17, 2019).

that "**good is good enough.**" I am glad to see that the soon-to-be-published research supports that philosophy. I also believe it supports the values of *cooperation and collaboration* in medicine instead of competition and isolation. These two ideals for which Living Medicine strives to include in its approach are encouraged between physician and patient, as well as between physician colleagues.

For many years, the concept of *wellness* has been the goal for those of us working in the health care field who are striving to see this "larger picture" and extract ourselves from the "disease-care industry." (Norm Shealy, MD[238] has been describing our current state of affairs in medicine with this term for over twenty-five years.) The deeper I went into what *true* healing was all about, the more I realized that, if wellness was our *only* goal, we were limiting ourselves. We all have corns or constipation or something—but I am much more interested in "holism." When we, as patients begin to assume responsibility for *our own* health, we will *have* to make changes. *Physically*, we may need to change our diet, exercise regimen or water intake. *Mentally*, we may need to change our attitudes. *Emotionally*, we may need to work with and understand our feelings. *Spiritually*, we may need to accept ourselves as spiritual beings. *Only then* will we be able to turn around and come back up from the dark place towards which we have been heading. *I have worked with many people who have conditions which they will never "cure," and they* still *live lives that are complete and fulfilling.* To illustrate, let me tell you about a friend and patient who is a perfect example of these Living Medicine principles. This patient/friend is currently a seventy-three-year-old woman who, despite experiencing her first stroke twenty years ago, was able to go to a movie with me three weeks after that episode! Most people (including some physicians) have *never* believed what she has lived through. When she was eighteen months old, she climbed a ladder up to the second-story window of her parents' house where, when she saw her mother's face, she let go of her hold on the ladder and fell

---

[238] Shealy, C. Norman, MD. Third Party Rape: The Conspiracy to Rob You of Health Care, 1993.

headfirst into a tar bucket, fracturing her right clavicle and right elbow. Her arm kept her head from going into the tar. However, her right kidney was severely damaged. It had to be removed and, until she was eight years old, she was on dialysis or had tubes in her kidneys which drained into gauze pads when she was not on dialysis. When the rest of us talk about our childhoods, she has nothing to say because she spent most of hers in hospitals, and her schooling was with tutors. By the time she was eleven, she had developed pyelonephritis (infection) in her remaining kidney, which then fibrosed (scarred) and left her with less than half of one kidney. She went through high school and college, then gained enough advanced training to work in neurophysiology and pharmacology. She had three miscarriages and one full-term pregnancy which, sadly, was a stillborn because of toxemia. She then had a hysterectomy at age 27 and bilateral mastectomies at age 39. Her second stroke occurred three years ago, in the same location as the first stroke, just on the *opposite* side. Nevertheless, she has continued to live her life *fully*, facing each of life's challenges as they come her way, and there have been *many*. Recently she said to me: "Illness has never defined me, and I refuse to let it do so now, even with this *new* bump in the road [her second stroke]."

This patient/friend has taught me many lessons, not the least of which is to pay attention to what she tells me! She knows her body and how it functions *for her*. She also knows what she can and cannot handle in the way of medications and procedures, as well as what life situations are good for her and which are not. She learned much from her mother and the caring doctors who paid close attention to her responses. *Her mother never treated her as an invalid and never put up with what she called a "pity party."* Whatever the situation was, they dealt with it with as *little* drama as possible. *She always thought of herself as a healthy person* because **she focused on what was right** and working *well* in her body—*not* **on what was wrong with it**. If something was suggested in the way of a therapy which she knew was *not* right for her, she stood her ground. She sometimes got answers from her dreams. She is *not* reckless, *nor* does she dismiss her physicians' recommendations. Rather, she is thoughtful and clear about her needs in *all* aspects of her life, including her therapeutic interventions. She will never be totally "well," yet she has found a way to live her life to its *fullest*. She has always been "aging into health," because *her focus is on Life*, not *on any disease or part of her life that is not* fully *functioning*. SHE HAS A CHOICE, as we all do. The difference is that *this patient truly lives her life understanding this fact and acts accordingly*. I encouraged her to write the story of her remarkable journey, which she finally did![239]

I know of many other people who are living with some chronic disease, yet are shining examples of a Living Medicine life, and I am sure that we all know people who are doing the same. *When we focus on Life* instead of *an illness, or any part of our life which is not well, we often spend our Life Force looking for what we* don't *have.* In so doing, we may miss out on what we *do* have and on Life itself, which is the *real* Healer. If we choose to live our lives abundantly, our choices will be filled with *living* energy, hope and light, and we can then "age into health," as my patient/friend is doing so well. Of course, there will be difficult and dark times in our lives. However, we *will* live through them and *not* get stuck, *if* we **stop trying so hard *not to die* that we forget to live**! **"Aging into health" can** then really **be boiled down to *living* until we die**. In my mind, to age in any other way simply makes no sense!

As our house of Living Medicine is built, it becomes a personal and very individual *dwelling place.* It helps us look at and remove obstacles in our lives that have created problems through the years. It creates a solid and stable foundation, balancing science and art. It helps us accept into our living space the conditions in our life's journey that we must face. Doing so moves us into the nurturing and nourishing aspects of ourselves, taking us even deeper into our very core. *It is in this core that birth and death, as well as the connection between the conscious and the unconscious minds, truly dwell.* It helps us accept the reality that assimilation and elimination are essential to our

---

[239] Woolf, B.I. (Bobbie). By No Coincidence, 2018.

health and well-being, and that *rest is vital.* It helps us acknowledge that play is important to create *balance* within our living space and to look at and identify the way our dwelling place fits into our external environment.

Our house of Living Medicine *can be a tent or a million-dollar mansion.* It **is what each one of us** *chooses* **to create and build.** This Living Medicine home helps us *not* neglect or back away from storms or difficult situations that arise in our lives. Instead, it helps us look at them for what they *mean* in our experiences. It encourages us to "try" (in the Cayce context of persistence) not to kill, destroy or hide these experiences. Rather, it encourages us to furnish and decorate our home with the day by day, moment by moment experiences of Life. In this way, they become part of our cellular structure in this physical body as well as in our eternal soul. As we look at our dwelling place, our home of Living Medicine, we see that it has been built on solid ground. The foundation is also solid—it is balanced, stable and true. Our house fits into the environment and is part of the neighborhood. It is a welcoming place, *not* a battleground. The grounds are well-cared for, and it *feels like* home.

I have a lifelong friend who is almost a hundred years "young," who is aging into health. Even though her life has not been easy, she has built a home of Living Medicine as *her* dwelling place. It is light and airy. Although very small, it is correctly built ecologically. As a two-year-old, she had hepatitis (which almost took her life), then suffered from bouts of malaria for many years. She had a learning disability. Yet, in her teenage years, she was able to move to a different culture and adapt quite well. Although school was hard for her, she did achieve an advanced degree. Her pregnancies and births were hard. She had mumps as an adult, followed by a mumps infection of the kidneys and ovaries, as well as kidney stones. She survived cancer twice, as well as a devastating divorce, through which she lost her business. She then *reclaimed* her life and created a *new* business that is now giving her the opportunity to *truly* achieve her life purpose. In her home of Living Medicine, there are interesting art objects that are displayed according to what seems appropriate to her. I like to go and visit her. If you ask her about her philosophy of Life, she will tell you that she truly "*lives* in gratitude," *not* that she has an "*attitude* of gratitude." There are many times when her finances are so low that she must borrow money to pay her bills, yet she views this fact as a *passing* thing. Life, she says, has been good to her, and life is *still* good.

Each one of us can build our own *house of Living Medicine*. No two will be alike. Life's experiences, both painful and joyful, can be used to give *each* home its own character. Even those of us who are in our nineties or who are 100 or more are *still* building, because **our dwelling place is a *living* thing**. Being a living thing, we will always find new materials with which to continue to build and improve our physical and spiritual homes. These building materials can come from many sources, one of which has evolved from stem cell research. Because stem cells are *living* cells that *create life*, they are a way to approach the treatment of disease that focuses on the *energy* of Life. Also, as our body *continuously* recreates itself (ninety-eight percent of it yearly,[240] *not exactly* "every seven years" as previously thought[241]), *our own* stem cells are *always* available to us.

This concept about stem cells became real to me when I was talking to a lady who had been a patient of mine for many years and had asked me about stem cells. As I talked to her, I became aware of a new way of working with them. In 2009, at a meeting that Rose Winters, Executive Director and CEO of The Foundation for Living Medicine, and I had with Roger Nocera, MD,[242] we learned about the stem cell research he had been doing in Costa Rica.[243] He said that some interesting results had emerged from that research. The research protocol

---

[240] https://www.npr.org>story>atomic>tune-up>how>the>body>rejuvenates>itself (July 14, 2007).

[241] www.snopes.com>Fact>Checks>Science>does>the>body>replace>itself>every> seven>years (April 30, 2018).

[242] Nocera, Roger M, MD. Cells That Heal Us From Cradle To Grave: A Quantum Leap in Medical Science, 2012.

[243] www.cellmedicine.com.

that he had been using was always the same, meticulously carried out in every detail. However, in this one laboratory, there were some stem cells that acted differently. They were healthier in the petri dish and, when they were transplanted into the patient, they exhibited more life energy than other stem cells. Nobody could figure out why this was so until Dr. Nocera decided to just sit in that specific lab and watch what was going on. What he found was that one specific lab technician in the lab approached the stem cells he was working with differently. Dr. Nocera observed that this particular lab tech *talked to* the cells he was working with and may have even prayed with them. Whatever that lab tech did, he was really engaged in the life and health of those stem cells and appeared to *really* care about them. Dr. Nocera's conclusion was that lab tech *loved* those cells, and *it was his love that made the difference in how those stem cells acted*. After relating this story to my patient, I said to her: "What's wrong with us? Why do we think we have to take stem cells *out* of our body, give them to *somebody else* to care for and love and then put them back *into* our body? Can't we connect with them while they're still *in* our body and let them know that we love them and that we can take care of them and help them grow?" This, of course, does not mean that there may not be times when help may be needed from the *outside*.

This concept reminds me of a time when my oldest daughter (Analea) was about three years old, and I was watching her try to tie her shoelaces. I went over to try and help her. She looked at me, stomped her little foot, wagged her little ponytail and said: "I'd 'wather' do it mine ownself!" I backed off, as she continued to struggle with her shoelaces. Finally, she stopped, looked me straight in the eye and, in a very commanding voice, said: "If you 'evo heped' me, 'hep' me now!" I think that is the way it is with stem cells. I think, at **first**, it's good to **make an effort to heal ourselves**. In other words, we need to first work with *our own* stem cells to let them know that we love them, that we know they're there to help us heal, then give them some direction as to what *we* think needs to be done. Despite our best efforts, however, that self-healing approach is sometimes not quite enough to give us the results we are seeking. **When we *do* need help from the outside,** I think it is good to **accept it and work *together* with it,** as we engage in our healing process. My patient understood what I was saying. She began working with her own stem cells with joy and delight and found that she was healing faster. *She was able to heal her knees enough* on her own *in this way to complete her planned pilgrimage along the Camino de Santiago trek in Spain!* I have had other patients also be able to visualize and work with their own stem cells in a loving, caring manner who have created amazing results in their lives as well.

The reason that diseases may be overcome by the growth of our *own* stem cells (or another's stem cells injected *into* us[244,245]) is because Life *does* overcome death, just as Light *always* overcomes darkness. *The life of the soul goes on after the body dies, no matter what your ideological concept of that process is.* If you ever have a chance to go to Carlsbad Caverns in New Mexico, you will have an experience of light overcoming darkness. In the deepest part of the main cavern, the guide will turn off *all* the lights, and the darkness will be as palpable as black velvet. When the guide strikes *one* match, the light from it is enough to dissipate *all* the darkness. This example, in a way, is reflective of stem cell treatment, in that **with the proper placement and nourishment of stem cells, *all manner of tissues* within the body *can be regenerated and regrown*.** This kind of treatment is truly an example of how Living Medicine works with the Life Force to bring about *true* healing. Two very different cases demonstrating this possibility come to mind now.

Every few years, The Foundation for Living Medicine holds a conference called "The Best Medicine of Tomorrow, Today." It is really a "think tank" for physicians and researchers who are pioneering new approaches to healing to get together to present their ideas to each other and discuss them. At the most recent one in 2018, Dr. Ann in-

---

[244] Riordan, Neil H, MD. Stem Cell Therapy: A Rising Tide – How Stem Cells are Disrupting Medicine and Transforming Lives, 2017.

[245] www.ncbi.nlm.nih.gov>pmc7033303.

vited the physician who taught and certified her in stem cell therapy, Dr. John Young,[246] to speak. At the conclusion of his presentation, Dr. Ann asked him to share his experience of using stem cell therapy with his daughter (Kathryn), their fourth child, born with "full-blown Down's syndrome." Dr. Young stated that the physician who took care of his daughter in the hospital after she was first born told him and his wife: "From looking at her genetic profile, she will likely be sick most of her life and need to take a lot of antibiotics." With that news, they took her home and loved her, just as they had done with her three older brothers. When she was old enough, she was placed in a special education program at her school. "Upon starting Pre-K, we were told that our daughter was highly uneducable, that she had very good social skills, but *nothing mentally*. Initially, I learned to do stem cell therapy so I could treat the *four torn ligaments in my own knee* in an effort to avoid knee surgery. I used *screened* umbilical cord stem cells obtained from a reputable stem cell bank that *only* stores products from normal births. It worked! I was back playing tennis, *without* surgery, within three months of my injury! I then ran across some research from Germany where stem cells from sheep had been given to Down's syndrome children which resulted in raising their IQ about twenty points. That's when I decided to treat Kathryn with the same kind of stem cells I had used to treat my own knee." At the time of his lecture at our conference, Dr. Young had treated his daughter three times over a period of one year. At the end of each one of those treatments, he said he had gotten a call from Kathryn's teacher asking what had changed in her care. "What do you mean?" he asked the teacher. "Within a few days after the first injection [IV], the teacher said Kathryn had started to say *words* that the teacher could clearly understand. After the second injection four months later, the teacher reported that Kathryn was able to use words in *phrases* that were now accurate and understandable. After the third injection four months after that, Kathryn began to speak understandably in *full sentences*! At

---

[246] Young, John D., MD. Beyond Treatment, 2014 and www.youngfoundationalhealth. com.

that point, the teacher said that my daughter was now 'highly educatable' as far as the school was concerned and felt that she had a bright future." Dr. Young's story is truly an example of the importance of doing our "due diligence" as physicians in terms of researching the *science* behind holistic therapeutic techniques. In being willing and open-minded enough to "think outside-the-box" like Dr. Young did and using the Life Force options available to us as Living Medicine physicians, *true* healing really *does* become possible!

The second case is quite different, and *equally powerful*, as it involves using stem cell therapy successfully in an *energetic* form. It all started when Dr. Ann returned from her stem cell training with Dr. Young in mid-2018. She had really wanted to learn stem cell therapy because of the large veteran population where she lives in a rural community in southern Arizona. She had immediately seen the need for this kind of regenerative medical therapy in that population due to the extent of their combat-related injuries. A stumbling block arose, however, when Dr. Ann could not obtain malpractice insurance to cover her doing stem cell therapy in Arizona except to treat arthritic joints. Even for such limited use, including stem cell therapy increased her malpractice premium significantly. In addition, like most holistic therapies, this treatment is *not covered by medical insurance* because it is labeled as "experimental," even though there is *valid research* to support the efficacy of it and other non-mainstream therapies. After a year of fighting this losing battle to help her patients with *actual* stem cell therapy, she began to look for other options. That's when she was introduced to HALO biophotonic therapy. She read the research and heard the *inventor*, Michael Thomas's *own story* of how this amazing technology had *twice*-saved his life,[247] first from stage 4 leukemia in 2009 and later from stage 4 idiopathic NASH (non-alcoholic steatohepatitis)[248] in 2017. With the first diagnosis, Michael was told he was a "dead man walking" and should already be dead. With the

---

[247] www.halomultiverse.com.

[248] https://www.niddk.nih.gov>symptoms-&-causes-of-NAFLD-&-NASH (for overview); click View or Print All Sections for full article).

second diagnosis, he was told he had "maybe four months" to live if he received a liver transplant. Since mid-2019, Dr. Ann has used this *efficacious, cost-effective light therapy* successfully to accomplish with her patients (including some of the veterans) what she could previously only envision being achieved with *actual* injections of umbilical cord stem cells. A few of her cases (with photos) are discussed in one of the videos on Michael's website. She is particularly happy to have this *energetic* form of regenerative medicine available for her *chronically* ill patients, especially those who also have significant environmental illness and are hypertoxic. Why? Because a landmark 2005 study conducted in part and published by the Environmental Working Group[249] showed that *two hundred eighty-seven chemicals and pollutants in the human umbilical cord blood* of ten infants born in August and September of 2004 in U.S. hospitals "cross[ed] the placenta as readily as residues from cigarettes and alcohol! This is *the human 'body burden'*—the pollution in people that permeates *everyone* in the world, including babies in the womb." This umbilical cord blood was found to harbor "pesticides, consumer product ingredients and wastes from burning coal, gasoline and garbage." Needless to say, Dr. Ann now feels quite thankful that she is *not* injecting *actual* umbilical cord stem cells into her patients, not to mention being able to save them the significant cost of doing so. Clearly, stem cell therapy is a valuable addition to the physician's therapeutic toolkit in whatever form it is done (visualization, injection of *actual* stem cells and/or energetically stimulating *the body's own* stem cells with biophotonic light therapy). Research like the EWG study simply points us in the direction of how we can *improve on* what is already an extremely promising healing therapy in the twenty-first century that can help us *all* truly "age into health." I have repeatedly said: "If someone doesn't pick up and run with what I have done, said and written, it doesn't amount to a hill of beans." Thank goodness I have lived long enough to see people pick up the hill of beans!

---

[249] www.ewg.org>body-burden-the-pollution-in-newborns, July 14, 2005.

In the fall of 2006, *The Arizona Republic* featured an article about genetically-altered cells that had helped bring two men with *metastatic melanoma* back to health.[250] Although it represented early research, it showed promise. From the point of view of Living Medicine, the following statements made in that article are relevant (bold is mine):

> *"It's not like chemotherapy or radiation where, as soon as you're done, you're done,"said Dr. Steven Rosenburg, lead researcher and the [National Cancer Institute's] surgery chief. "We're giving **living** cells, which continue to grow and function in the body. We can take a normal cell from you or me or any patient and convert that cell into a cell that recognizes the cancer. After these cells are grown, they can then be injected into the patient and, as **living** cells, [they can] protect the body against the cancer cells."*

This type of research takes the Life Force and *enhances* it, so that **Life itself can overcome illness**.

Another type of research being conducted at Duke University works in a similar way by using genetically-modified polio virus. The researchers are using it to stimulate the body's own immune system to overcome the deadly brain cancer *recurrent glioblastoma*, which can double in size every two weeks. Once this form of the virus has been injected directly into the tumor, it attaches to the surface of the cancer cells and begins its attack. This is what jumpstarts the body's own immune system to finish the job. Researchers believe that *this secondary immune response is the most important part of the treatment*, as it is this response that starts to break up the tumor. CBS's *60 Minutes* program has been following the journey of the doctors conducting this research and their medical-pioneer patients for the past

---

[250] Arizona Republic, "Gene Trial Cures 2 of Cancer," Sept 1, 2006.

five years.[251,252] Results as of the last update showed that twenty-one percent of the sixty-one patients treated to date were still alive after three years on this experimental treatment, compared to four percent of patients treated with standard care. As a result, new clinical trials have begun using this approach to treat other solid tumors like breast cancer and melanoma.

With these two research findings in mind, as well as the awareness that we truly *do* create the body in which we live with our thoughts and our emotions, we can look forward to healing at an even *deeper* level that revolves around *living,* as the next two examples illustrate so well.

Another form of working with Living Medicine is the work of re-generating tissues that Robert O. Becker, MD (1923-2008) did in the mid-1980's. In his landmark book,[253] he explains and describes the regrowth of tissue (*entire* limbs and other body parts) by using *directed, low-voltage electrical currents* like the electricity that runs through each nerve in our body. This book opened a whole new possibility for healing to the world, the field of **energy medicine.** Dr. Becker's research became very real for me after meeting and becoming friendly with one of his neighbors who became interested in his work. We had several extensive conversations, one-on-one, during which she told me the following story about her sixteen-year-old son. Even though I do not recall the names of this mother or her son, I have never forgotten the story she told me.

One day, while mowing the family's lawn, a blade from the lawn mower came loose and cut off the tip of the index finger of this young man's left hand, just below the nail bed. His mother became very alarmed and suggested they go to the ER immediately. Her son replied: "Why don't we try what Dr. Becker has been talking about and see if I can grow it back?" His mother decided to go along with her

---

[251] Pelley, Scott. *60 Minutes,* March 29, 2015.

[252] LaPook, Jon, MD. *60 Minutes,* June 26, 2018.

[253] Becker, Robert O. and Gary Selden. *The Body Electric: Electromagnetism and the Foundation of Life,* 1985 and 1998.

son's idea, so she dressed the wound and stopped the bleeding, which gave her son some relief from his pain. He then began concentrating on his finger regrowing and, for several months, they just watched and waited. Sure enough, little by little, his finger began to regrow, including the nail bed and fingernail! They watched it regrow for six to eight months. Then, one day, the young man's mother noticed that her son's finger had stopped regrowing. Her son's response was: "I know. I stopped regrowing it on purpose because I don't want to be drafted! [This was the era when young men were being drafted to go to Viet Nam.] I think if I have this injured finger, they won't want me in the army!" **The use of Life energy to create and regenerate tissue reflects one of the fundamental tenets of Living Medicine.** This medical model is *so* much more hopeful and promising than the *conventional* one. I found it ironic that this young man used a *Living* Medicine approach to avoid the act of killing in the larger, global sense.

One other powerful example needs to be included, I think, to illustrate the power of the mind and how effective it can be when used for healing. Much like the story of my patient (Susan Kramer), Joe Dispenza, D.C. managed to heal himself from six vertebral fractures (T8-L1) that he sustained while competing in the Palm Springs triathlon in 1986 at the age of twenty-three after he was struck on his bicycle by an SUV traveling fifty-five mph. The T8 vertebra was more than sixty percent collapsed, and its shattered bone fragments were pushed up against his spinal cord. This meant that were he to try and stand up, those fragments would be pushed deeper into his spinal cord, and instant paralysis from his mid-chest down would result. How Dr. Dispenza *fully and completely* healed himself from his devastating injuries is a true *conventional* "medical miracle," as described in his own words that follow[254] (bold and caps are mine). **In the world of Living Medicine,** however, as I have seen demonstrated time and

---

[254] https://www.healyourlife.com/how-i-healed-myself-after-breaking-6-vertebrae (May 23, 2014).

time again by patients like Susan Kramer and Bobbie Woolf, **any-thing is possible**.

> *Maybe I was just young and bold at that time in my life, but I decided against the medical model expert recommendations* [from his surgeon and neurologist]. *I believe that there's an intelligence, an invisible consciousness, within each of us that's the Giver of Life. It supports, maintains, protects, and heals us every moment. It creates almost 100 trillion specialized cells (starting from only 2), it keeps our hearts beating hundreds of thousands of times per day, and it can organize hundreds of thousands of chemical reactions in a **single** cell in every second—among many other amazing functions. I reasoned at the time that if this intelligence was real and if it willfully, mindfully, and lovingly had such amazing abilities, maybe I could take my attention off my external world and begin to go within and connect with it—develop a relationship with it.*

> [W]hile I intellectually understood that the body often has the capacity to heal itself, now I had to apply every bit of philosophy that I knew in order to take that knowledge to the next level and beyond, to create a **true** experience with healing. And since I wasn't going anywhere [and] I wasn't doing anything except lying face down, I decided on two things. First, every day I would put all of my conscious attention on this intelligence within me [his Physician Within] and give it a plan, a

template, [and] a vision with very specific orders[...]then I would surrender my healing to this Greater Mind that has unlimited power, allowing It to do the healing for me. And second, I wouldn't let any thought slip by my awareness that I didn't want to experience. **At nine and a half weeks after the accident, I got up and walked back into my life—without having any body cast or any surgeries.** *I had reached* **full recovery.** *I started seeing patients again at ten weeks and was back to training and lifting weights again, while continuing my rehabilitation, at twelve weeks. I discovered that* <u>I was the placebo</u>*. And now, almost 30 [now 34] years after the accident, I can honestly say that I've hardly ever had back pain since.*

As we look at the lives and stories of these *ordinary* people who have healed themselves in *extraordinary* ways, it is important to put this information into context within *our own* individual lives. If we accept the reality that we have within us the power to heal *all* our ailments, we must also accept that doing so may *not* be what *our* soul's path is destined to do *right now*. Another way to understand this concept is this: we can all listen to and accept the reality of the music created by an operatic soprano and may long to be able to sing like that ourselves. However, *our* reality may be that the best *we* can do in the musical talent realm is to barely carry a tune! Just like we cannot all be operatic sopranos, **not all of us have the capacity to heal ourselves in *extraordinary* ways.** As physicians, our job is to offer our patients *all* the options we possibly can that are unique to *each* person's individual case or situation, *as well as* give them a glimpse of how patients (such as Susan, Bobbie and Joe) have been able to work with *their* Physician Within to produce *their* extraordinary results. Because our life path is unique and individual to *each* one of us, perhaps the healing path that is best for a *specific* patient (or even ourselves) *right now* may be a more conventional one, because they (or we) have specific lessons to learn from *that* path. Our job is to help the patient (or ourselves) find the *best* option for him/herself among *all* the choices available and then allow the Physician Within *each* of us to do the healing work to the best of each of our individual abilities. **What is *not* helpful on anyone's healing path is to be made to feel like a failure** (by ourselves or others) **if we have been unable to accomplish the extraordinary results that others have produced on *their* healing paths.** The truth is, healing from a common cold is an extraordinary thing, no matter what methods are used to do it! The ordinary does not always *have* to be extraordinary. **Doing one's best (in *any* situation) is *always* good enough.**

Our house of Living Medicine is not only our *actual* physical dwelling place, it is also a metaphor for the home where our soul dwells while on the earth: our physical body. One of the things about our body is that we cannot just move out of it at will and build a new one; not in *this* lifetime, anyway! *We must learn to dwell within this structure that we have both inherited* and *created.* Just like we *can* rebuild and/or redecorate our physical dwelling place, what manifests in our body is *also* the result of our choices and decisions. In the words of Stephen Covey[255]: "I am what I am *today* by the choices I made *yesterday.*" The people or thoughts and emotions that live with us in *both* of our dwelling places have helped build them. In *both* instances, though, *we* are the ones responsible for how *each* of them comes together. We might move away from either of them for a while, as in taking a vacation *or* while we are dreaming *or* when we are in altered states of consciousness. What we have created in *both* of them, though, is what we live with, and *both* of them ARE us. In looking at this amazing body in which our soul dwells, then, we must consider how karma and grace have helped to build it.

---

[255] Covey, Stephen. The 7 Habits of Highly Effective People, 1989.

As previously stated in the chapter five summary, my journey in medicine has included learning the Edgar Cayce material. Throughout this second edition, and especially in chapter five, I have given examples of how my understanding of this material has influenced the way I practice medicine. What follows is a deeper discussion of some of this material. I think it is especially important to understand in some depth Cayce's concepts of karma and grace in order to better appreciate the discussions that follow this information.

I remember a lecture given by Hugh Lynn Cayce many years ago entitled "Where Karma Ends and Grace Begins,"[256] which I have summarized from the handout that he gave us of that lecture (capitals, bold and italics have been used for emphasis, and my comments are in brackets). He defined *karma* as *our* memory *and* *grace* as *God's* memory. He said the concept that "karma is *just* memory" represents a profound statement. We humans remember good *and* bad, as well as our creative influences *and* our destructive influences. God, being the Essence of Goodness, remembers the good. **Goodness recreates itself**, but badness or **evil self-destructs**. If karma is *our* memory, what Hugh Lynn seems to be saying is that, as *we* remember goodness, it moves us from the Law of Karma *into* the Law of Grace. As long as we remember the hard times—our weaknesses, the things that we have done wrong or the way others have wronged us—we continue to feed "bad" karma [and thus continue it]. *If we stop feeding the memories of the hurts and the pain that we have sustained, they no longer exist.* "Good" karma has, within itself, the ability to create *more* goodness. **The bad self-destructs, the good self-perpetuates.**

Karma is the law of cause and effect and, if we look at this law as hardships to be faced, we continue to perpetuate a difficult and hard life. However, if we can understand the really beautiful opportunity we have been given in this lifetime to accentuate the manifestation of the "fruits of the Spirit," we will bring peace within ourselves *and* among humankind. Edgar Cayce says that a karmic debt is not [*just*] karma

---

[256] www.edgarcayce.org>holistic>health>database>where>karma>ends>grace>begins.

between people *or* karma with an *individual* person. Rather, a karmic debt has to do with *relationships* between people. *It is* [us] *meeting ourselves in relationship with another person.* If karma is *our* memory, then we are working with the *memory* of our relationship with another person. A karmic debt is one that we ourselves have that is being worked out [in the *relationship*] between ourselves and another person. The thoughts [we *individually* think] are the food upon which the soul [or relationship] feeds. We can continually feed negative karma by the negative thoughts that we think, *or* we can constantly feed our soul [*and* our relationships] with the good, creative and healthy thoughts we think. *All* personal relationships are part of a pattern, and we continually "meet" ourselves as we interact with each other. **Each soul pays for *its own* karma.** The following statements help us understand these aspects of karma and can be interpreted from a "bigger picture" perspective in light of it:

- **What we create in the earth plane must be met *and* corrected in the earth plane.** It cannot be corrected from the disembodied realm.
- **Only those you love may hurt you**, as they are the ones with whom we have karmic patterns that must be *constantly* corrected, because it is a *living* process.

How can we change the Law of Karma into a Law of Grace? **We come into this life with deep-seated karmic patterns**. We may have created in past lives a tendency to be jealous, to be angry, to look for contention and strife or to be consumed by self-pity. **We can change whatever our *specific* weakness is that we are born with.** It takes hard work. It takes a *lifetime* of work to change these tendencies. It takes prayer, meditation, working with our thoughts and feelings and understanding our relationships. **As we do this,** with God's help, we move under the Law of Grace. **These [karmic] patterns then become only *urges*** within our being, instead of an all-consuming pattern. In this way, a karmic *drive* [or pattern can] simply become [just] an *urge*. [Dr. Ann informed me that Bert Hellinger has demonstrated another way of transforming these patterns using the family constellation work he originated, the outcome of which is "to restore the order of love." He founded this approach after WW II to help people in Germany deal with and *truly* heal from "survivor's guilt."²⁵⁷] *If we create our relationships with* constructive *influences, we move under the Law of Grace.* In order to do this, **there are spiritual laws to follow.** As we work with these concepts in our relationships with other people, we begin to move into and operate from the Law of Grace. **We can thus learn about, experience and come to know the Divine because of what *we* manifest in our relationships with others.**

Edgar Cayce gave us the following *Seven Steps on the Path from Karma to Grace*:

1. **Choose according to your ideal.** Setting an ideal [*an individual's* ultimate goal or life purpose] is central to this work, and the ideal is on a physical, mental and spiritual level. It [must] be [a] *living* [goal or purpose], which means that the steps toward that ideal *can* be and *probably should be* always changing. [If you have your ideal and you work diligently towards achieving it, you can go through *all kinds* of other things in life, and you will not get off track.] We need to identify our *individual* ideal and separate it from ideas. **Ideas keep people apart, ideals bring people together.**

2. Act according to [your] ideal in line with the spiritual laws that we, as individuals, *currently* know and understand. **The only way we can make *our* ideal real is to do the best *we* can [in each and every moment].**

3. **Be creative, in the *little* things that you do as well as [in] the big things.** Find different ways of expressing and doing [*simple*] day by day actions.

---

²⁵⁷ Hellinger, Bert. Many offerings (in multiple languages) from www.amazon.com

4. **Give up criticizing and condemning ourselves and others**. [Feeding] our negative emotions [only makes them] grow. If we stop feeding them, they dissipate by themselves.

5. **Be not hurt by harsh words.** When somebody says something to us that we take as being harsh or critical, we can activate self-pity and self-condemnation. The harsh words cannot hurt us unless we take them [in] and *let* them hurt us.

6. Let peace enter your life and the life of everyone that you meet. **Pursue peace.** Peace does not descend upon us. We can pray for peace and long for peace. [However,] **if our *actions* do not create peace in our relationships with other people, there will be no peace**. Only as our actions and our thoughts work with [dwell on] peace with [our] fellow human beings will there *be* peace.

7. **Forgive yourself and others as God forgives us.**

Our house of Living Medicine is *constantly* being created out of the *balance* between karma and grace. *This is the brick and mortar that holds this structure together.* It is how we have *lived* our life, how we have related to the world around *and within* us, and how this balance (or lack thereof) has manifested in the flesh of our very being, which is our body. The **cells of our body not only carry our genetic code, they also carry our soul pattern.** *That* is how each one of us can be *uniquely* different, yet profoundly the *same*.

While all of Cayce's seven steps from karma to grace are important, the ones I want to emphasize here are the first and second ones; the ones that distinguish the difference between our *ideals* and our *ideas*. Explaining this using the following example has helped me understand this difference better, and I hope it will help you in this way also.

Let us say that the shared *Ideal* that most of the major religions can agree on is "God is love." The *manmade ideals* that each of these religions comes up with to achieve that Ideal, however, is *each* religion's *idea* of how to accomplish that Ideal. It is these *ideas* that separate different religions and are usually the basis for their disagreements with each other. Sometimes this happens to the point of killing each other over them (e.g. the lives that were lost in India when my parents were there with Mahatma Gandhi due to the partition of India in 1947 between the Muslims and the Hindus). When we use this same analogy in relationship to our *individual* selves, the shared Ideal of *all* humanity is to live a life that is creative and moving forward towards the Light. As long as each of us is striving to do that in our own *individual* ways (according to our own *individual* ideal), we can move through a lot of darkness and get over a lot of hard stuff, because we will not be drawn to investigate those dark places. On the other hand, if we focus on the things that take us *off* track from our *individual* ideal and/or our shared Ideal (or take our eyes off of either one for too long), we are likely to get into trouble and become "stuck in the mud" of the *ideas* that took us off track. This is how we lose our opportunities to move forward with *our own* ideal to achieve the *shared* Ideal. A more specific application of this concept in medicine can be explained this way: when we stay on track with our *individual* ideal, we may *go through* or *experience* diseases; however, we will not *become* those diseases, because **it is not necessary to** become **the disease** to achieve our *individual* **ideal as we move forward towards achieving our** shared **Ideal. Though it is sometimes necessary to go** *through* **illnesses or diseases,** it is *not* necessary, however, to *become* them!

If those of us who are trained as physicians and those of us who are aware of the Physician Within can allow *our* Divine nature to manifest in such a way that Light and Life, joy and healing are the energies that motivate *us*, then the Divine energies *can and will* work with the hardships, the diseases, the pain and the problems we face in *our own* lives. They will *also* assist us to help our patients face these things in *their* lives as well. These life events then have the possibility to be experienced as *blessings* instead of enemies. **Even death itself can be transformed into being recognized as part of the Circle of Life**, instead of being held as a devastating tragedy that sometimes keeps us (and our patients) *stuck* in grief.

When *our* ideals as physicians LINE UP with the *shared* Ideal of *all* humanity, life is just easier and can flow better. Doing so allows us to swim *with* the current in a river *instead of* against *it*. There may be times, however, when our CHOICE is to swim *against* the current. We may choose to do this for a specific reason. For example, if our life choices have been taking us *away* from our ideal, we may have to swim *against* the current to get ourselves back on track. **Understanding this principle is what can bring us *peace* in those moments of choice instead of feeling continually conflicted, even when we make the "right" choice.**

Another example: there may be times when a piece of furniture, such as a couch, is worn out or no longer fits in our living room and should be removed. Similarly, a benign uterine fibroid, or even a cancer, could have grown and now is something that just simply needs to be removed. We, as physicians, can be helpful in taking out or getting rid of that *specific* structure. By the same token, there may be someone or something that has moved into our home and completely taken over and disrupted the functioning of it. Metaphorically, this could be pain, cancer, some chronic illness or even another human being. The role of the physician in this situation might be to help facilitate the removal of that person or thing. The physician also needs to make sure that, when whatever has moved in is *gone*, there is not an empty space left in the house that would *re-attract the same problem* (or something even worse) into that empty space. As Living Medicine physicians, we also need to be ready to receive and/or create some new *living* energy to reclaim that empty space, so we can teach our patients how to do this in *their* lives. I teach patients how to do this using their dreams. I tell them to *first* make the *best* decision they can *on their own*, from all the information currently available to them. I then suggest that they think about their decision as they go to sleep, asking the Divine to give them a dream to help them know if this is the *best* decision for them *at this time*. I tell them to *expect the answer from their dream*, if they have one. I also let them know they can call me for help with their dream interpretation, if necessary. For most patients, this approach works very well. Most of the time they learn to do this process of decision-making all on their own without my help.

Dr. Ann helps her patients with their decision-making in other ways. One way is that she teaches them about what she calls the **"Rule of Three."** She learned this **principle** from Gay Hendricks[258] in 1992, and it goes like this: If something happens *once*, it can just be a "random" act in the Universe. If that same something (or a similar something) happens a *second* time, it's time to pause and ask yourself: "Hmmm – could this be a pattern in my life?" If it happens a *third* time, that something most likely *is* a pattern—like three points on a data graph makes a straight line and needs to be looked at and dealt with as a pattern. Another way Dr. Ann teaches her patients to make their decisions is to learn to use their body's own intelligence (their Physician Within). She teaches them this concept as she uses neural kinesiology[259] in her practice to evaluate their autonomic nervous system (ANS), the "automatic" nervous system that keeps our organ systems functioning without *conscious* direction on our part. The exam is called a "biofeedback-enhanced physical exam," which Dr. Ann uses *in addition to* her standard physical and osteopathic exams. When her patients have healed enough to be able to truly sense their body's innate intelligence at the ANS level, Dr. Ann teaches them a *simplified version* of this exam that they can use for themselves any time they choose. Once they receive their body's information in this way, she suggests that they "sit with it, meditate on it, pray about it, ask for a dream…whatever it takes for you to feel in your body that *this* answer is right for *you* at this time."

No matter which way we teach our patients how to make *their own* decisions, as Living Medicine physicians we are partnering with our patients' Physician Within to teach them the principle of *self-responsibility*. This process can also be a reminder that our body's

---

[258] www.hendricks.com.

[259] McCombs, Ann, DO. "Neural Kinesiology (Autonomic Response Testing)," www.nonprotocolmedicine.com>new-client-information>new-client-information-packet, p.17-19.

symptoms on *any* level are just the way it is trying to communicate with us until we can hear its message. When we respond to whatever that message is in a way that treats the *underlying cause* and not just the symptoms, *true* healing can happen, and the symptoms will not usually return.

I was talking to a friend recently who said that she had been struggling with emotions she felt were the result of frequent hurts that she had been subjected to from other people. She told me her way of responding was to build up what she called "a hard heart," which in her words "had made my heart become stone." She had been thinking about this issue while hiking. She looked down and saw a stone on the ground that was perfectly heart-shaped. She picked it up and went through a ritual in which she built a little altar on the path on which she had been traveling. She then put the stone in the middle of that altar and did her prayer work, offering up the stone and asking that her heart be softened. She prayed to be awakened to the compassion and love that she wanted in her life and had been afraid to allow in. When she finished, she went home feeling lighthearted and free. The next morning, in her meditation, she worked with her guardian angel and said something about having placed the stone in a special place along the path. She began to describe the stone when the angel spoke to her and said: "If you want to, you can go back and pick that stone up again and let it be your heart. You can do that. You can do that at any time." In that moment, the woman realized this was exactly what she had started to do. *In her mind*, she had gone back to the path and picked up the stone, reliving the things she thought had created the hardness of her heart. She grasped what her guardian angel was saying to her: "You can leave the stone where it is and go on with your life *or* you can go back and pick it up and continue to carry it with you as your heart of stone. *That's your choice.*" My friend chose to leave her stone on the path and continued with her life, awakened to compassion and love. *If we do not replace our negative thoughts with positive and constructive ones, the negative ones just come back in.*

My friend understood the importance of words. Even in television ads, the **words matter**. For example: I have been listening to advertisements about medical treatments and have become aware of how important their words are. In their television ads, they state: "We *only* treat cancer (or whatever else is being advertised). We don't treat anything else." Somehow, as I listen to those words, I wonder how the *patient* fits into these treatment programs. I know that these treatment centers pay a lot of attention to the individual person. I know that they are very aware of the importance of *treating* the individual person. However, *their words* belie the importance of the *patient* and, somehow, *make cancer more important than the individual patients themselves.*

As we live in our house of Living Medicine, there are times when we pull back from the world, and it becomes a dwelling place of quiet and inspiration. It is the place where we draw from *within* ourselves whatever wisdom and understanding *we* need to go on with life. It is also the place where we derive the hope and strength to face what is going on in the world *outside* of us, as we look at and strengthen the world *inside* of us. These times of withdrawal and inspiration can be caused by some painful event that has happened *or* because our soul is just saying: "I need time with *me* in this house, so I need to now draw back from my *outside* activities for a while." There are also times when our soul says that we are becoming *too* complacent or *too* content with the way things are. In these times, our soul may really be telling us "it's time to grow." That may mean that it is time for someone or something to move in with us. *Consciously* invited or not, we must find space for the *new* energy. This growth process could be a new relationship, a new concept, a new thought, a new theology, a new emotion or something that is not part of the house that we originally built. Nevertheless, the new energy moves in, at least for the time being. Our choice then becomes to accommodate, make comfortable, make useful *or* make the decision that this energy is no longer welcome, and it is time to move out. There may even come a time when we are *forced to grow* because of some traumatic event that blows off the side of our house. When this happens, we must adjust to whatever it is in the world around us that has imposed itself upon our house, turning it into a crisis situation. When that happens, we have a *different* choice to make: we can either pull back into a corner of our house and disappear *or* we can accept the challenge that comes from having this whole new situation forced upon us. In choosing the latter option, we have several other choices: we can either rebuild the wall the way it was; reconstruct it in a *different* way, doing whatever is necessary to accommodate the new vision that has been forced upon us; *or* move out altogether and find *new* accommodations better suited to us. From *these* options, we can then create the opportunity to GROW *because of* the crisis.

There are other times we grow because we have looked out and seen a *new* vista. We have seen something that is so beautiful and so engaging that we know we *must* open the windows of our mind to this thought, to this *new* dimension of consciousness. This awareness allows us to see beyond anything that we have encountered before—vistas of land, air and sea or whatever it is that has opened itself to us. This is one of the ways grace can enter our life, filling it with love and beauty. It may be some specific illness that has caused us to stretch our vision beyond our previously limited window space, and now shows us a world that is so much greater and so much more beautiful than we had before. Or, perhaps, the world we now see out there is so needy, it draws us to that need. Then, in the process of dealing with and involving ourselves with that need, a *true* healing can take place. It may be that the disease process itself is now a member of our household; yet, we may find that our life is so much richer because of it. Such a guest can even help us expand and beautify our life, *despite* the hardships. It can also cause us to *endure*, so that we no longer feel restrained and restricted by the four walls that we originally created. There will be times when we will be drawn into this new vista, whether it is because of the very beauty of the new landscapes we see and a need to experience them *or* a need to be involved in some aspect of life that may be painful or difficult. **As we venture out,** the fact that we have built our home of Living Medicine on *solid* ground allows us to stretch beyond its boundaries and grow, because we know we *can* and *will be able to* come back to our *solid and stable* foundation.

Dealing with a *personal* illness may move us into areas of pain or discomfort that are beyond anything that we have experienced before. The knowledge that **our home of Living Medicine is where the Physician Within us dwells, allows us to understand a perspective of** *true* **healing that only occurs** *from the inside out.* Because of this perspective, the Physician Within us understands *why* the illness arose, and *the best way to work with it*, so that *true* healing can happen. There are also times when some *other* problem might come to stay and remain with us for the rest of our life. This problem then becomes *part* of our life and part of our *ongoing* life story. There are also times when a disease is something that a person can *so* incorporate into their life that it enhances and makes them a stronger and better person. Franklin Delano Roosevelt was able to do just that with post-polio syndrome, and then go on to become president of the United States during the Great Depression!

Some of the people I know as *truly* healthy beings are people who have a chronic long-term illness that they have been told they will *never* overcome—yet it has *not* stopped them from living their lives *fully*. They respond to it like a tree when it is putting its roots down and comes upon a huge rock. *The tree has two options*: one is to put all its energy into breaking that rock apart and going through it; the other is to extend its roots *around* the rock and incorporate the rock into its root structure and then extend its roots deeper into the earth. The latter choice makes the tree more stable and solid and better able to withstand the storms that come along in life. Then, if the tree is blown hard, its root structure has the rock incorporated right into its very being and becomes even more beautiful for having the rock there. In this metaphor, the chronic long-term illness is the rock, and the tree's roots are the healing Life Force that encompasses that obstruction and transforms it. On the other hand, if the person with the chronic long-term illness chooses to deal with it by putting all his/her energy into breaking that rock apart and going *through* it (assuming the tree's roots manage to break the rock apart), *what happens to those broken pieces?* I wrote an article[260] about this principle. I think it is worth including here.

> *In the mid-1980's, Harmon and June Bro, along with Bill and I, led a group of A.R.E. members on a trip through China. We were on a boat on the Li River and stopped at a small dock where local people were selling goods. I purchased two beautiful china plates with dragon designs in vibrant colors of green, turquoise, purple, yellow and red. When we got home, Bill and I ate our dinner off those plates almost every night.*

> *Years later, I was washing one of the plates when it slipped out of my hands, fell to the floor and broke into five large pieces. I really did not want to throw those pieces away. They were still beautiful and reminded me of visiting Bali and seeing the walls of their temples with pieces of beautiful ceramics built into the walls. So, I placed these five broken pieces in my meditation garden. They and other beautiful ceramic fragments live among my flowers to this day. I heard that, in Japan, if a piece of china gets cracked or damaged and the owner still sees in it great beauty, it is called Wabi*

---

[260] McGarey, Gladys Taylor, MD. "Treasure the Broken Pieces," Venture Inward: The Magazine of the A.R.E. and the Edgar Cayce Foundation, December 2014.

Sabi[261] and the damaged part is considered to add more value to it.

As the years have gone on, I have begun to see these and other subsequently broken pieces of china as a metaphor for the way I practice medicine. When we look at our lives, we can see how all things are connected, and that connectedness creates a pattern which produces a living, beautiful aspect to our lives. I have watched some of my patients whose lives were so difficult and so broken, whether by disease or life circumstances, form a connection with the Physician Within themselves. Their lives take on an added beauty and, despite their brokenness, they become shining examples for the rest of us.

As previously mentioned, Franklin Delano Roosevelt was a good example of a person who lived a *complete* life, even though his body was broken. If each one of us will make the effort to look at the pieces of *our* life which have been broken and find in them the rare beauty which is unique to *us*, our Life Force can then imbue *our* broken pieces with that beauty and help us to create continuity. **Let us be very careful about what we throw away**. *Some of our most painful experiences hold the brightest treasures*, as we look for and find the beauty in each aspect of our life. As we joyfully incorporate the *broken* parts with the *living* parts, we become one—*whole once again*—and life is good! This concept, I think, is an extension of a proverb that Edgar Cayce often quoted, which has always meant a lot to me: "Grow where you are planted."[262] So, let us take the *broken* pieces of our

---

[261] Kempton, Beth. Wabi Sabi: Japanese Wisdom for a Perfectly Imperfect Life, 2018.
[262] www.quotemaster.org.

lives that still hold great beauty for us, and let the Christ Consciousness (which is our Life Force) transform them, so that our lives are enriched, and we become *truly* whole.

As we age, we find more and more broken pieces in our lives. As we discard those that no longer serve us, we can find places for those that bring us joy, beauty and light and can then *age into health*. We no longer need to focus on *anti*-aging—we can *embrace* our added years, wrinkles and all! I have discovered that wrinkles never hurt until we begin messing with them. From the *inside*, they feel perfectly smooth! As I touch them on the *outside*, they also feel smooth! It is *only* when I look in the mirror or at a photograph of myself that I *see* the wrinkles, and they allow me to see myself the way others see me.

Inevitably, there will come a time when the soul needs to move out of its house of Living Medicine and go on. It can be that the person has lived a few hours or a hundred or more years in their earthly home. At that time, the person gathers into their soul the experiences they will take with them into the future. The thoughts they have had, the emotions they have felt, the things they have done, the people they have seen and the relationships they have had—all of these are now part of *their* karmic pattern or part of *their* soul memory. They gather this all together and are then ready to walk out the front door and meet whoever or whatever is waiting for them as part of their future. This is called death...*and* **Life *goes on***. The structure or the body that is left behind is now an empty shell. Because there is no longer life *within* it, it will, because of its very nature, crumble and die. In biblical terms, this is what is meant by "dust to dust."

My birthplace is Fatehgarh, India and in these latter years of my life, I have found myself drawn back to India quite frequently, and *not* just to visit. I have had work to do in India as well as in many other parts of the world. Because the concept of Living Medicine is so real in my life, I find that the experiences I have *each* day help me understand the *true* meaning of this concept at a deeper level. As I mentioned previously, my parents went to India in 1914, right in the middle of World War I. My oldest brother was three months old when they left New York to go to a land where they knew no one. They did not know the language, they did not know the customs, and I doubt they had ever met a person who was East Indian. They went, despite the fears and doubts that arose, *knowing* that there was work that needed to be done in India for which, somehow, they were qualified. Being physicians, they understood that India needed the love and caring that physicians could bring to her. Their deep abiding faith in a loving, compassionate God carried them across the Atlantic Ocean, where German submarines were infesting the waters, to a life that was to become a shining example of true love and commitment to their children and to the countless lives that my parents' lives touched. Their lives, for me, manifested the reality of Living Medicine. Not once did they become the many diseases that they lived through, which included sunstroke, amoebic dysentery, smallpox, malaria, malnutrition, abscesses and a host of other maladies. They faced each difficulty knowing that it was part of their life's journey and, with God's help and a love for life and their fellow human beings, they would get through these difficult times. When they began their work with the *children* of leper parents, they offered them a home filled with love and understanding. Each one of those children was moved out of *becoming* a leper (that is, becoming the disease that their parents had) and into becoming just people who worked at whatever they individually chose as their life work. In observing my parents do their work with these children, I learned that **the point of life is *not* to just stay alive, it is to stay *in love with life* in all its forms**. Just like God uses imperfect people to do His perfect work (e.g. Abraham, Moses, Joseph and the Apostle Paul, to name just a few), we too must make a *paradigm shift* from believing that we have a karmically-burdened body with a soul to understanding that **we are ALL *living* souls manifesting in bodies with karmic patterns called diseases**. As Carl Jung once said: "The most painful issues in life can't be solved...they have to be outgrown,"[263] just as **our *old* ideas of people and diseases must be outgrown and *transformed* into a more empowering and truthful paradigm**. To me, **this is the essence and goal of Living Medicine**.

As I think about India herself—this land of my birth, this magnificent part of our world—which, for countless centuries has been invaded and conquered, had her riches stolen and her lands confiscated, I cherish that *she still lives*. When the Mogul kings came and conquered the whole country, the essence of India herself was activated from within. These kings activated their own creative energy and love, so that some of the most beautiful structures in the world were created by the great khans. Ultimately, Shah Jahan built the Taj Mahal for his wife (Mumtaz Mahal), and it is the most perfect example of *true* love in physical form. *The Taj Mahal, in all her beauty, represents to me the Divine Feminine in labor.* The magnificent dome is the uterus. On either side of this dome are the breasts, and the four phallic symbols stand guard. The great entrance is the opening through which the baby is born in a flood of water. This wonderful building holds a special place in my heart and in my life, because my mother went into labor with me at the Taj Mahal! I have no words to adequately describe how meaningful it was for me to be physically present at the Taj Mahal, at sunrise, on my eightieth birthday. I was blessed to return again in 2007 with some of my children and grandchildren.

The ebb and flow of life that is Living Medicine manifests in my life in *each* moment of *every* day that I am alive. *Each* of us has been blessed with the *same* opportunity to experience living Life in this way, *no matter what circumstances we were born into*. In our homes of Living Medicine, we will *all* step onto our own back porches and watch our loved ones create their own sunsets. Yet what *we* see of that sunset will be *our own* personal experience. No two people experience a sunset in the same way, just as no two people experience each other in the same way. By the same token, none of us experiences the *same* disease in the *same* way, just as each sunset is dif-

---

[263] Wilhelm, Richard (translator), Jung, C.J. (Foreword and commentaries by). The Secret of the Golden Flower: A Chinese Book of Life, 2014 reprint of the 1932 edition.

ferent. We will all die and bring *our own* life, our days on this earth, to a closing sunset. **Our challenge is to *experience* our lives with *all* its joys *and* difficulties**. When we die, we will not die of cancer or any other disease process. Instead, we can view this culminating experience like my daughter (Analea) did: "after *experiencing* cancer" (which could also be any other disease process or life circumstance).

As individuals, it is only when we look honestly at our difficult places and our shadow side that we can *truly* feel the love and joy of our true nature. **Peace only results from dealing with conflict in an open and honest way, with a willingness to look at *all* sides, in order to deal rationally with the conflict and arrive at a solution for the good of *all* concerned.** The only way we can have an abundant life is by allowing ourselves to *truly* live and *truly* love, instead of shying away from life or choosing to sleep through it.

William Sloane Coffin, in his wonderful book entitled *Credo*,[264] has two quotes I would like to share here:

> *It's hope that helps us keep the faith, despite the evidence, knowing that only in doing so has the evidence any chance of changing.*
>
> *Martin Luther was right: "God can carve the rotten wood and ride the lame horse."*

With these two quotes in mind, I look at the future of medicine with great hope. The *evidence* that we are faced with is that of a broken system. **The *solutions* for correcting this broken system** are fragile. They **must deal not only with the *symptoms*, they must *also* deal with the *underlying cause* of the sickness, if the solutions are to be effective.** When we look at the evidence that presents itself, we can become discouraged and continue to look for ways in which we could patch up the tears in the fabric of the system itself that

---

[264] Coffin, William Sloane. Credo, 2004.

leaves us vulnerable and still broken. However, with hope and faith, we have a chance to change the evidence and create a system that is whole and strong. **If God can "carve the rotten wood and ride the lame horse,"** then, with Divine help, we can create a strong *and* loving health care system. *To do this, we need to change our focus from killing and destroying to living and loving.* **The paradigm of Living Medicine gives us the opportunity to do this.** We can take our God-given creative energy and focus it on life *and* living, *then* use the tools that have evolved in the *science* of medicine to bring the spirit of love, hope and healing back into the practice of medicine. The concept of Living Medicine allows us to understand that **it is Life and Love that are the Great Healers. To whatever degree we look at illness and disease as something that needs to be destroyed and gotten rid of, it is hard to come to grips with** *true* **healing. You can cure a disease and not heal the patient. You can also heal the patient and not cure the disease.**

I have been striving to create effective solutions to heal our broken health care system all my professional life as a physician. My early efforts to accomplish this task were previously detailed in previous chapters. Since that time (after Bill and I separated in 1989), I continued my pursuit of this goal through the formation of a not-for-profit foundation, first formalized in the early 1990's. This foundation has changed names several times, though the name that "stuck" and resonated the most with me, as *I* became clearer about *my* ultimate purpose (*my* ideal) on earth this time, is The Foundation for Living Medicine. We plan to move forward by creating my *global* vision, The Village for Living Medicine, a vision that I have held for over fifty years!

On May 1, 2009, a group of thirty-five physicians, many of them A.R.E members, gathered in Scottsdale, Arizona to pull together a "white paper" to send to the White House at the request of President Barack Obama. This information was then distributed to *many* like-minded groups to help him solve the national health care crisis at that time. All the doctors who came to that historic gathering had been actively involved in working to solve this health care dilemma as *in-*

dividual practicing physicians for many years. We called this meeting a "Gathering of the Eagles." We all shared the core belief that **effective health care must encompass BOTH the *art* of healing and the *science* of medicine**. We then created a structural framework which would lead to this paradigm shift in medicine. We based this framework on the concepts of the importance of the *physician-patient partnership* and taking *individual responsibility* for one's own health. We realized that to accomplish the task before us, we needed to address the question of *how to marry the* art *of healing with the* science *of medicine*. For all of us, this task required *a fundamental shift from a focus on fighting disease to the promotion of individual and community wellness*. It also required *an acknowledgement of the body's* innate *ability to heal itself* (the basic tenet of *osteopathic* medicine, which Edgar Cayce very strongly recommended) as well as *the importance of including love and spirituality in the healing process*. It recognized that **unconditional love is Life's most powerful healer** and **the perceived loss of Love (meaningful connection with others, including our pets, and/or the Divine) is our greatest health risk**. These basic concepts are what I had long been calling *Living Medicine*, which I finally *officially* identified as the paradigm shift that I wanted to manifest. To make them real in the world, and thus *instigate* this paradigm shift, we proposed to President Obama that it become **essential for *effective* health care delivery to *transform itself from a commodity "industry" to a "ministry" of human service*.**

As I have mentioned throughout this book, many of the principles of Living Medicine are based fundamentally on the philosophy and information that comes from my study of the Cayce readings. *Our culture has shifted its focus from personal responsibility for one's health to dependency on outside resources for our healing*. The concept that **the Physician Within *each one of us* is the being that does the *actual* healing** has not been considered part of the health care system since the time of Andrew Taylor Still, the founder of osteopathy and osteopathic medicine (1828-1917). As a result, *personal responsibility* for healing has not been well understood for almost a hundred and twenty years, since he founded the first osteopathic medical school in 1892, previously mentioned. Hippocrates (460-375 B.C.), on the other hand, known as the "father of medicine," is the one we can more accurately attribute being the "father of *modern* medicine," as he described in a *scientific* manner in his more than seventy books many diseases and their treatments, after detailed observations.[265] **As long as we as patients expect the Physician Without to do the healing, we will *not* be able to get to the *root cause* of our medical issues.** *To the degree that we continue to focus on fighting* diseases *instead of healing* individuals, *we will never really understand what the fundamental problems are in our health care system.*

In one of Edgar Cayce's readings, he said: "All healing, then, is from Life! Life is God!"[266] To understand Cayce's words, I believe, requires a paradigm shift in our understanding of health and healing. One of the reasons that the Cayce material is *so* complex is because *each* reading was given to a *specific* person at *a particular time*. It dealt with a *living* process, one that was *constantly changing* and *completely individual*. As students of the Cayce material, we need to accept the fact that, in Cayce's words, "all healing comes from One source."[267] That Source is the Life Force in each one of us. *A surgeon can suture a laceration, but only the patient can heal the wound.* **The patient does the healing.**

As we feed our physical, mental and spiritual being with food that brings life and healing, we will then begin to know that correcting this broken health care system is going to require more than a financial fix. **Each one of us must take responsibility for our life choices and acknowledge our *interdependence* with each other and the whole earth.** For Dr. Ann, this principle has been defined

---

[265] www.britannica.com>biography>Hippocrates.

[266] www.edgarcayce.org. Reading 2153-6.

[267] www.edgarcayce.org. Reading 2696-1.

and explained best in the following way by Stephen Covey[268] (bold and capitals are ours):

> *On the maturity continuum,* **dependence** *is the paradigm of* **you**—*you take care of me; you come through for me; you didn't come through; I blame you for the results.* **Indepen-dence** *is the paradigm of* **I**—*I can do it; I am responsible; I am self-reliant; I can choose.* **Interdependence** *is the paradigm of* **we**—*we can do it; we can cooperate; we can combine our talents and abilities and create something greater together.* **Dependent** *people need others to get what they want.* **Independent** *people can get what they want through their own effort.* **Interdependent** *people combine their own efforts with the efforts of others to achieve their GREATEST success.*

Once physicians and patients *truly* understand this principle and these distinctions, they will begin to see that it *requires THIS KIND of teamwork* and a deeper understanding of the *living* process to be able to *begin* to get a handle on how to work with our broken health care system and *transform* it. As I previously said, if someone doesn't pick-up and run with what I have done, said and written, it doesn't amount to a hill of beans. Many people are now working towards this paradigm shift, for which I am truly grateful.

The Edgar Cayce physical readings give us a foundation upon which we can build a *living*, dynamic health care program for our country, both locally and nationally, then globally and inter-nationally. The Foundation for Living Medicine is currently seeking to collaborate with other partners to further this paradigm shift in medicine

---

[268] Covey, Stephen. *The 7 Habits of Highly Effective People*, 1989.

and implement whatever it will take to bring about this transformation. I plan to spend my hundredth year (and every other moment that Life grants me *after* this year) doing all I can to bring these changes into being...and I even have a ten-year plan! Dr. Ann is equally committed. She learned the following **principle** at the age of twenty from another of her brilliant teachers[269] (who learned it originally from Thomas Kuhn, the author who introduced the term "paradigm shift" in his landmark book, *The Structure of Scientific Revolution,* [270] named one of "The Hundred Most Influential Books Since the Second World War"[271]):

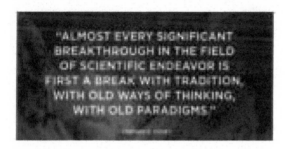

It is her prediction that this second edition of *Living Medicine* will eventually be found on some equally prestigious list in the future! However, we would both be content to have it be used widely as THE textbook that brings about this next paradigm shift in our beloved chosen profession...***Living Medicine.*** She would also say, in the famous catchphrases of *Star Trek*'s Mr. Spock and Captain Jean-Luc Picard, may we both "live long and prosper" enough to "make it so....[and let us] boldly go where no one has gone before! Things are only impossible until they're not. Captain's Log, Stardate [2020]....Engage!"[272]

---

[269] Covey, Stephen R. The 7 Habits of Highly Effective People, 1989.

[270] 50th Anniversary edition, 2012; originally published in 1962.

[271] Times Literary Supplement, 1995.

[272] Roddenberry, Gene. Star Trek: The Original Series, 1966 and Star Trek: The Next Generation, 1987.

About the Author

Dr. Gladys Taylor McGarey is a medical pioneer and visionary. She was born to medical missionary parents in the jungles of India a century ago, in a place and time that filled her childhood experiences with imagination about what medicine could be. As the only female cofounder of the American Holistic Medical Association in 1977, she has become affectionately known around the world as the "Mother of Holistic Medicine." The year 2020 marks her one-hundredth year on planet Earth, and she continues to usher in the next medical paradigm shift, Living Medicine.

Made in USA - Kendallville, IN
1224810_9781949001938
01 14 2021 0919